The

Personal Trainer

Companion

The Complete Guide to ALL Aspects of the Fitness Industry

by

Michael Jonathan Rocco

For Suni- if we just believe!

Contents

Welcome...5

Set Up and Marketing...7

Chapter One: Personal Trainer Certification...12

Chapter Two: Sports Nutrition Consultant...113

Chapter Three: Advanced Personal Trainer Certification...157

Sample Forms...222

Sample Exams...224

About The Author...282

Index...285

Welcome

Greetings! In this book, you will find information designed to prepare you for a rewarding career in fitness. In America, the importance of physical development has increased dramatically; there has never been a better time to engage in this industry. As a fitness professional, you will become a respected advisor, trusted confidant, an important member of your community, and in many cases, a friend.

Whether you work for a club or start your own business, having the proper credentials will award you the qualifications needed to establish yourself in this growing field. On your own, you can make anywhere from $45-200 per hour depending on your reputation in the industry. In the beginning, it is recommended that a trainer offers rates of $45-65 per hour or $25-35 per half hour sessions. It is also beneficial to offer packages to your clients so you can receive full payment up front and secure client relationships. There is a great deal of creative freedom in this area. You can design packages to your liking (i.e. 10 sessions for $399).

As a fitness professional, you are responsible for client safety, providing accurate information and good conduct. Your clients will undoubtedly speak volumes about you to friends and family (referrals are integral to a trainer). Likewise, they will surely spread a campaign of misery if you offend them. Always try to be calm and polite at all times. Even if someone insults you or your pet sawdust, remember to respond in a professional manner. It is also highly recommended that you take a CPR course in the event of an emergency. You can take a basic course in your local area (usually the fire department offers this) or you can obtain information online.

Finally, make sure to have each client fill out a health questionnaire and release form before starting any program. You will find sample forms towards the end of the manual. Feel free to print out and use these forms and routines

in your new business.

Set Up and Marketing

Setting up your own business is not as daunting of a task as you might think. There are different procedures, depending on the state you live in. For instance, in the state of New York, a new business owner must first register their business name. This is commonly known as a D.B.A. or *Doing Business As* title. You can pick any name for your business that has not already been taken in the area. Think of something catchy that has relevance to your field. You can find out where to go by visiting your county civil service website or by searching the government section of the yellow pages. It usually doesn't cost more than $45 and it only takes a few minutes. Next, you must obtain a tax identification number. There are state websites such as O.P.A.L. in New York that now let you apply online for free. This will enable you to write off your business expenses each tax quarter. Try to keep all records and receipts organized in separate files.

Once you have completed these steps, you can decide where you want to conduct business. Some people are independent contractors in established gyms, while others open a storefront location. The most popular occurrence for a self-employed trainer is traveling to your clients homes. While all three of these methods are beneficial, renting space is the most expensive. The overhead alone may not be worth the risk to someone just starting out.

In either case, it is important to purchase an insurance policy in the rare event someone gets injured. Though it is unfortunate, it will give you some degree of relief knowing you've been covered in such an event. There are various choices of insurance policies. Chances are, the moment you make your business legal, different companies with find you! A basic policy will average about $200 per year. This will cover you for up to $1 million dollars. Even with a policy, you should have each client sign a waiver sheet during their initial consultation. Sample forms have been included in this manual for you to use. Beyond insurance and liability forms, don't be afraid to refuse training to anyone who sends you negative vibes. It's your business and you can train whoever you want.

Marketing your business can be fun and inexpensive. Here's a list of ideas to help launch your campaign:

Flyers/Postcards: they're dirt cheap to have made or you can design and print them yourself. Post them everywhere that's legal! Great locations include residential homes (you may need to pay for postage), apartment complexes, university campuses, doctor/dentist/chiropractor offices, libraries, supermarkets, and in local health food stores.

Business Cards: a must in this industry. You can easily print them yourself or have them made. They cost around $20-40 per 500 cards in most places online. Just Google "business cards" and you'll see. These can be distributed amongst family, friends, colleagues, coaches, and your medical providers. Always keep a stack in your wallet!

Website: there is no denying the power of the internet for advertising and selling products. You can easily build a free website from Bravenet or Tripod, but once you've built up some momentum, it makes a HUGE difference if you pay $10-30 per month using web hosting services from Yahoo! and many others. It helps to insert meta-tags on each page of your site. This is the HTML code that is your actual site. Ask your host how to insert title tags, keywords and descriptions to your pages. More and more, people are linking to other websites. This helps major search engines place you in better spots. Finally, there are still reputable companies that offer inexpensive opt-in email campaigns. This means thousands of registered people will receive your ad. Setting up a good website takes time and patience, but once it's operational it'll be well worth the effort. Also, take advantage of social media sites including Facebook, Twitter, Instagram, and YouTube- they're free and thousands of potential clients will have access to your posts and videos.

Local Papers: you can place ads in local town papers such as Carrier Trader or whichever you have access to. Start by running smaller ads each week and increase ad size and placement once your phone begins to ring.

Placemat Advertising: have you ever been to a diner and noticed a placemat stuffed with local business ads? They are cheap and effective.

Radio/TV: many places have *Public Access* television stations where you can advertise cost effectively. There are also independent/college radio and satellite stations that will accommodate your business needs. Check your TV guide and local college campuses for contact information.

Movie Theaters: if you're a daring type, you can place your ad on movie theater screens in your area. All of the major theaters offer this option, though it may be costly. Of course, imagine just how many people will see it before the movie starts.

CHAPTER ONE:

PERSONAL TRAINER CERTIFICATION

Motivation

Mind Over Everything

This section is not as much about your client-it's really is about *you*. Each year, many people earn credentials as fitness professionals, only to end up quitting within months. Personal training is more than routine reps, sets and body fat percentages. Helping people improve their lives takes courage. It takes compassion. It also requires determination when business is slow or when a client is ready to give up. If you don't believe in yourself, your clients won't believe in you either. The following information is important and should be taken seriously. I am amazed by how few books in this field delve into this subject matter. The technical knowledge you'll acquire in this book will mean *nothing* if you don't feel good about yourself.

Once you feel confident, you'll be in a better position to help others. Always remember:

As a fitness trainer, your number one objective is to inspire. Period.

You have the right to be happy and have everything you want. How come there are those few who seem to have it all, when the majority live paycheck to paycheck? Some people have close relationships with their husbands, mothers, sisters, cats, etc., when others eat alone every night. There are 17 year-olds who have Irritable Bowel Syndrome (a certain young author suffered from this at that age), while there are senior citizens who have cast-iron stomachs. Is it all genetics and luck that ultimately decide our fate? In my humble experience, I've learned this much and I'll try to be delicate: THAT'S COMPLETE BULLSHIT! Contrary to popular belief, most people who have what they want (be it money, relationships or whatever), attained these goals, regardless of what their grandparents felt or how they grew up. Sure, there are those who inherit wealth (although most rich people didn't), but that doesn't mean they're happy and have what they have. This reminds me of the age old philosophical dilemma, "Which came first, the chicken or the egg?"

Do people have good attitudes first and then get what they want or do people get what they want and form good attitudes? Let's figure it together, shall we?

Depending on your point of view (which is a huge part of this subject), a person who has been kicked around their entire life, may develop a poor outlook. Then again, we've all heard about the rags to riches cases, where people who start out impoverished and unhappy, end up building financial empires and feel great. In contrast, there is also the positive and energetic young woman who always wanted to fall in love… only to have her heart broken several times. She started out with a cup half full or even completely filled up, but slowly poured it out in stride with every abusive man in her life. These opposites can become confusing for the unconscious mind, which is arguably the biggest factor in what we attract.

You've undoubtedly heard of the mysterious unconscious mind and its magnetic pull in our lives. Put it this way- if you regain control over this so-called monster, you'll have full control over everything else. This is not necessarily in relation to positive thinking either (you can think whatever you want, but if you don't believe it, it probably won't matter). The problem with the unconscious mind, is that most people don't know how it all works. Here's how I look at it:

Picture your brain as an office, fully equipped with a computer and file cabinet. Every time you volunteer a statement or thought, you are using your *conscious mind*. For instance, if you were to say "I'm so ugly," you are basically typing that statement into your writing program on your PC. From there, that text is automatically printed out as a new file and indexed into the file cabinet- your *unconscious mind*. That's really it- your unconscious is an unbiased storage facility. It doesn't care whether your files are good or bad; it simply stores them as records. Now, let's suppose you were to say "I'm beautiful!" Here's the deal- if you already have an epic stack of files stating the opposite, this new printout is just one piece of paper filed among an army of insecurities. Does this make sense? Here's another example:

DAUGHTER

Hello?

MOTHER

Hey, it's me.

DAUGHTER

Hi, ma. How's it going?

MOTHER

(sigh) Alright, I guess.

DAUGHTER

What's the matter?

MOTHER

Nothing. Never mind.

DAUGHTER

What? Just tell me.

MOTHER

No, it's just that... we haven't heard from you much lately.

DAUGHTER

Mom, I know. I've been so crazy with work and school...

MOTHER

Whatever, it's no big deal.

END

Oh, but it is a big deal, isn't it? It's not just what *you* declare that becomes a file; how you respond emotionally to the world around you also gets stored. You've been absorbing external stresses since day one. The dialogue above is common, as is the feeling of guilt associated with disappointing loved ones. The daughter isn't wrong for living a busy life. Yet, the last thing she wants to do is hurt her mother. In contrast, mom has her own file cabinet jam-packed with a mountain of "the good old days." She was once her daughter's hero, best friend and protector. Now, she feels replaced and rejected. You might say "Yeah, but her mountain of positive files about her daughter should outweigh the one or two negative ones, right?" *It's not so much the statements that matter, but the feelings underneath them that count.* Everything that you say, think or do, as well as how others affect you, are being written up into files… including the feelings associated with the event. As frightening as this may seem, you have control over this.

Again, if you tell yourself "I'm beautiful," but have hundreds of contrary files stored, you won't believe these words. Now, if you were to think of something positive (i.e. the concert you're going to this evening or the X-mas gifts you're opening tomorrow morning), that may help put you in a happy state. Once you feel good and excited, stating "I'm beautiful," will have an entirely different result. Let's do an experiment. Make sure you complete each step before proceeding to the next one:

STEP ONE

Close your eyes and think of something about yourself that is bothering you (something you would like to change). It can be anything- you're broke and feel like a loser or maybe you feel ugly; it can be anything close to you.

STEP TWO

Good. Now, open your eyes and state the opposite of what's bothering you, i.e. if you feel like a loser, say "I am a winner!" Make sure to say it aloud. Ready? Begin!

STEP THREE

Ok, all done? You may be experiencing negative feedback- you want this statement to be true, but you don't really mean it. This is normal. Since feeling positive is the best way to connect a statement to a belief, let's shift gears for a moment. Think of something that makes you feel happy. Take your time- this should get your energy up, so find something fresh. For example, if there's a movie opening tonight that you've been anticipating for weeks and you're going to see it, followed by a shopping spree at the mall, you'll probably be as excited as a 12 year-old boy at the arcade. Or, maybe the thought of improving your life by reading this book will get you into a better frame of mind. These are just my examples- you must create your own. If you can't find anything, think of your niece or German Shepard. Crank one of your favorite songs and dance like freak (it's hard to be upset when you're doin' the robot dance in your dining room). Be creative- the sillier, the better! If you still don't feel up to speed, I would suggest taking a walk outdoors and come back to this later on. We all have triggers- you'll find yours. Be patient and don't be hard on yourself if this doesn't work right away. Once you feel good, you'll be ready for the final step.

FINAL STEP

Now that you're feeling elated, make that positive statement again! Really get into this one- you're your best cheerleader, so don't be shy! Get pumped; if you trust me and do this, you won't be disappointed. Seriously, don't be afraid to shout it out. ARE YOU READY? SET? GO AFTER IT:

"I <u>AM</u> A WINNER! I <u>AM</u> A WINNER! <u>HOLY CRAP, I REALLY AM A WINNER!</u>"

How do you feel now? Hopefully, you went step by step and didn't just skim through this exercise. The idea is to associate positive feelings to a firm statement, so that you'll believe in what you're filing into your unconscious storage cabinet. The more you practice this, the more proficient you will become. It takes time- be patient. You spent years learning math in school and you didn't even care about that (no offense to any math teachers... *especially Mr. LaGuardia*). Give yourself a chance! If you don't lose 15 lbs in two weeks, don't panic- cause that's a file too!

The more feeling attached to a file, the thicker it will be. Also, the more files you create, the higher they will ascend. Having said that, there's still a huge stack of negative files- how can you catch up to those? Well, if you want to compete with them, you can (but it may take a while… and it'll be difficult). I have a better way. "Uh-oh, he's got another experiment." You guessed it!

All you'll need for this exercise is a piece of paper and a pen. The idea is to think of a memory (this should be something from your past that hurt you). If you were bullied in school, you may recall certain incidents that have stayed with you through the years. Maybe you have a memory of a humiliating event that led to feelings of inadequacy. Again, take your time- these are not the type of things that we reflect on often, so really dig deep into your soul. Did your parents divorce? Did you get fired from a job you really worked hard at? Perhaps you are overweight and have bullied yourself for a while. In any case, write down as many of these memories or feelings as you can. It doesn't matter if you list thirty five things or just two. As long as your list has meaning, it's all good. Here's a sample list:

1. In sixth grade, I was afraid to go to school. It was my first year in junior high and I didn't have many friends. One eighth grader, Billy the Bully, used to make fun of me on the bus. Everyone laughed with him. I remember being scared and would sometimes walk home to avoid him.

2. The popular- rich kids didn't accept me, because I wasn't one of the originals... my family relocated to Terrytown when I was in fourth grade. I was made fun of on a daily basis, because I didn't wear the cool clothing. My grades suffered from being distracted and I felt stupid. Even worse, one kid wrote in my yearbook and said "See ya next year... if you make it." This hurt a lot and despite my improvement in grades, I always felt shy around certain students.

3. I damaged my knee playing soccer when I was nineteen. I had surgery a few times, but still have a lot of pain. I've tried everything, but nothing helps.

I'm depressed and can't even play soccer anymore... which is my greatest passion.

4. When I was seven, I really wanted a video game system, but my parents told me that they couldn't afford it. I heard that all of the time growing up and now I'm always struggling financially. I feel inferior to my friends and can't seem to figure out what I'm going to do.

5. My first love broke my heart. No, actually, he ran it over with his truck. I know I wasn't perfect... sometimes I became angry and called him names. When he cheated on me, it nearly destroyed me. I haven't been able to carry a relationship since.

Once you have completed your list, read it once or twice and set it down. This may be very difficult for you or you may feel some relief just by writing these thoughts. Next, on a separate piece of paper, create positive replacements for each of your items. For example, if you were told that you were ugly as a child, replace it with "I am beautiful, inside and out. I know I believed those kids and added to their insults over the years, but I absolutely love myself just the way I came." Don't be afraid to defy your first list- be strong and let each one of these bad memories know who's in charge. Here's a sample list of the new files:

1. I was a great kid. I was young and sensitive and that was a good thing! Billy the Bully was wrong for what he did to me... he was just a mixed up and frightened little boy. Although I never deserved to get picked on, he and others have NO power over me now. In fact, the past doesn't even exist, unless I allow it to. I'm very strong and compassionate.

2. Those brats missed out on becoming friends with a great kid. I had so much to offer them. I also know that they were just children and didn't know any better... they learned their cruelty the same way I learned to ride a bike. Some of them are probably great people and would feel terrible if they knew the impact they had on me. Others may not be so nice today, but that's there problem to deal with, not mine. I'm VERY smart. A stupid person couldn't write lists and improve themselves. I love learning about new subjects and take every so-called failure as a lesson.

3. I have control over my body! I tell it what's up, not the other way around. My doctor can worry about it; that's what he gets paid the big bucks for. I'm going to heal. I have the power to heal my pain and I WILL heal my pain. Stress and tension have only exacerbated my symptoms, if not cause some of them. With patience and determination, I will play soccer again. I'm taking my body back! I'm taking my body back!

4. It's no wonder I'm having such difficulty with money and jobs. All I ever heard about growing up was "It's too expensive," and "We're not rich, ya know," and "Rich people are selfish and shallow... money isn't that important." ALL NONSENSE!

Money is great! Making money is easy! Money works for me... I don't work for money! Finances aren't intimidating to me anymore, but fun. I like making money and money likes being made. I can buy whatever video game system I want. I have the same right to wealth as any other person on Earth. I deserve to be wealthy!

5. He was wrong for cheating on me. I am a human being. Yeah, I wasn't perfect all of the time and I wish I didn't say certain things, but I am a good catch and he doesn't have power over me. There are a lot of great guys out there that will understand and appreciate me, for better or for worse... that's maturity and that's real.

**** I deserve to be happy. I forgive myself for not being perfect through the years. I am a good person. I AM a good person. I forgive those who have hurt me (not just for their benefit, but for my own peace). I love who I am today, flaws and all. I am* *beautiful, smart, funny, warm, and energetic! I love my life! I can accomplish anything and everything that I choose! I love my body... in fact, I'm going to kiss my own arm right now... MWAAHHH!!!*

OK, there's just one last thing to do: TEAR UP OR BURN EACH ONE OF THE NEGATIVE ENTRIES ON YOUR FIRST LIST!!! STOMP IT INTO THE GROUND!!! You have successfully assumed control of your mind. Repeat this exercise as many times as needed.

Congrats! You just made an important step towards manifesting your potential. Now put the book down and go have a great night- you deserve to!

To Believe Is To See

When you were young, what did you want to be? I'm 99% positive you didn't go "I want to be a motivated, self-starting, team player... working in a cubical from 9-5:30 for some rich boss. Then I want to sit in traffic, come home, take a nap, eat a TV dinner, watch the latest so-called 'reality show,' go to bed, wake up early the next morning, and do it all over again for 30 years." If that's what you said at five, you wouldn't be reading this. When I was young, I wanted to be a rock star, a business owner, a superhero, a writer, a black belt, and a jewel thief (which meant an actor playing one). Guess what? I'm a successful musician, I have acted in stage productions as well as film, I've run successful businesses, I'm a superhero to my family, I'm obviously writing, I've earned black belts, but I never stole jewels (I never played a thief either, although the mob boss came close).

You may be wondering, "What made the difference for you? What gives?"

Glad you asked, but first a question for you- it may sound strange, but if you widen your scope, you'll appreciate it. Who are you? I don't mean your name or personality. Let me rephrase the question: *What* are you? We've been conditioned since the womb to except the "reality" we're wrapped up in each day. Real life for most folks is the crappy job, car problems, root canal without insurance, communication trouble in our marriages, rationing our grocery store funds, migraine headaches, family disputes, getting ripped off by a power seller online, son's doctor visits, etc.

Let's pause for a moment, shall we? Close your eyes (unless you're driving) and take a deep breath. Isn't it amazing how much we take our existence for granted? Don't worry, I'm not gonna turn sideways on you, but please hear me out. Look at your hands for a moment. Now look at the familiar scene around you. What is all of this? Perhaps it has occurred to you that *"WOW, I'M ACTUALLY ALIVE RIGHT NOW. SOMEHOW, THIS IS REALLY HAPPENING."* Try not to ignore this, because regardless of your personal beliefs, this experience is astounding. When you stop what you're doing and really think about it, isn't it just bizarre? *You're here right now.*

This isn't a dream (or maybe it is), but you're the observer in this picture show either way- the protagonist, if you will. Do you know what it took in order for your life to take place? (No, I'm not talking about the stork dropping you off.) Whether you're an atheist, Catholic, Muslim, biologist, or naturalist, the fact that we've adapted to our living environment is miraculous. The fact that there is a living environment for us to dwell, is nothing short of incredible. We can think, feel and reason, without any proof of what makes this happen. Psychologists will point to neurons and connecting webs in the brain, but they can't explain *why* it works, any more than we can explain fire. Sure, we have scientific codes and hypothesis that demonstrate how fireworks, but *why* does fire work? How about the light bulb? Thomas Edison was ridiculed and even laughed at during thousands of failed experiments (if they were failures at all). Are people laughing at him now? No. Do we understand why electricity works? I didn't ask how it works- technically speaking, he could have stuck a banana inside a foxhole and added shredded newspaper and BAM, THE LIGHT BULB! That didn't happen to be the formula, but I think you get the idea. Children always ask their parents "Why" for everything. Usually, we don't know what to say, other than "Because I said so," or "Cause that's the way it is." With all of our technology, routines and assurance that the sun will come up each day, we have no idea that we're experiencing an awesome miracle. Nothing is what is seems to be, even if we don't acknowledge this notion. Getting back to your picture show:

If this is all possible, then why do you have so many limiting beliefs about smaller attainments?

Is becoming a millionaire the grueling task we think it is? Your body is constantly working for you at every corner you turn, in ways you don't even understand. That's more challenging than making a fortune. It's just that we have grown accustomed to the "world" around us and form beliefs about how things are. There's a good story that may shed more light on this topic.

Years ago, there were two Mexicans who had decided to leave their home and find work elsewhere. Up until that point, they had never seen an automobile. They had absolutely no reference for a car in their minds. While walking along a dirt road, a pick-up truck stopped and the driver offered them a ride. They hopped on back and away they went. The driver asked the men where they were headed and they replied "to the nearest town." As they approached a village, the men decided to get off the truck… while it was doin' thirty miles per hour! They simply jumped off and rolled several yards down the street. *The freaky part is that they were uninjured.*

The point of the above story is that these guys had no prior experience with a moving vehicle, in relation to the laws of physics. They couldn't see the danger of their environment. They stepped off that truck, the same way we walk through doors. If someone could've put a camcorder inside their heads and witness what they actually saw, that person would win the Nobel Prize.

How we see the world, shapes the world.

A word of caution: Do not attempt to flee from a moving vehicle. Agreed? Cool, let's move on. We've all heard the expression "Seeing is believing," a logical deduction that governs most of our lives. I've learned that the opposite is true. When you truly believe something, to the point of knowing with all of your being, it will become a reality for you. This is not to say there won't be work involved, but you will undoubtedly live your beliefs. You already do. Maybe you believe in dumb luck:

Dave is lucky that his dad owns a business and he'll take over one day.

It figures- before I pulled up to this traffic light, there were no oncoming cars approaching. Now I have to sit here for another two minutes waiting for them to pass.

I didn't have a chance to play piano like that girl. Her parents bought her the best lessons possible and encouraged her to play. My parents didn't.

He's got better body building genetics than me. All he's gotta do is work out for twenty minutes a day and he'll be ripped. Not me... I'd half to work six hours at the gym for three years to look like that.

You can clearly see how conditioning our beliefs our entire lives can hurt us. Is it possible that everyone gets stuck at a light now and then, but some people don't get upset over it? I usually use traffic as an excuse to change the album I'm listening to. Maybe the person driving the nice car worked six days a week for twenty five years before they could lease it. I used to complain that my parents never bought me guitar lessons for my 6th b-day; I play in a successful band today. Are all of the good ones taken or are we *really* looking for the good ones? For the most part, we create our own circumstances. There are obvious exceptions- I don't believe that an infant attracts a kidnapper, because she feels vulnerable. Many babies do feel vulnerable and turn out just fine. Having said that, I believe that we are responsible for far more than we're willing to accept.

Think about your daily attitudes and how they may be altering your life. Start with today's thoughts and actions; did you spill a cup of coffee on the way to work? Did you turn it into an epic soap opera? Did someone snub you at the office and if so, are you obsessing over it? If possible, write these down. If you don't have access to paper and a pen at the moment, remember to come back to this later.

Now think of the things you want for your life and the beliefs you associate with them. For example, if you want to be a dancer, what thoughts do you connect with becoming a dancer? How long have you been thinking this way and most importantly, what feelings do attribute to these thoughts? Again, write them down, if possible. This will help you organize your thoughts and you'll also have a model to review when needed. Have fun!

Take a good look at your lists. Honestly, is it any wonder why your dreams have yet to manifest? These associations are the prime ingredients to the recipe of loneliness, poverty, poor health, and discord in America today. Imagine the ripple-effect we create with thoughts and feelings on a daily basis. Tension alone can compromise our physical and mental wellbeing, in addition to the "soul-food" we consume in an attempt to feel better about our lives. People use various means to compensate for their lack. Some resort to crime, others overeat, and so on. A good example of the power of association is evident in Emily's story:

After my divorce, I had spent three years alone and sick. Surprisingly, I didn't equate my stomach pain to the loss of my husband; I searched online for every known disease and was convinced that I had at least two of them. I don't recommend message boards if you're in pain! At one point, I found hundreds of people complaining of similar symptoms. These guys became my army of validation. I knew I had a serious illness. I was afraid to see a specialist at first, because there was no doubt in my mind I had some form of cancer.

When I finally conjured up the courage to see an urologist, I underwent a colonoscopy. After the results came back, the doctor spent all of five minutes with me. He said that there was nothing wrong with me, other than a nervous stomach. I couldn't believe it. "There has to be a mistake," I said. "I don't have cancer?" I remember his facial expression, one of familiar annoyance. "What about spastic colon or epididymis?" I was actually negotiating an illness with the poor man! "You can't have epididymis," he replied with a dry grin. "Only men can get that and even then it's uncommon." We then talked about my divorce and the stress I was under at work. It was becoming clear to me that not only did my husband and I split up, but I dropped playing violin after I started feeling pain. It was hard sitting upright for more than a few minutes, so I gradually spent less time playing music.

It's funny, but after I had left the doctor's office that day, I recall sitting my car for a while. I had such a sense of relief, but at the same time, I was still skeptical. He didn't even give me a prescription for the pain; he only recommended some chewable fiber tablets. Today, I'm engaged to a great man and resumed playing my violin. I feel terrific. I have always heard about the power of tension over the body, but I never thought it could cause such pain.

Emily's story isn't uncommon. After my second surgery, I also went on message boards and found tons of evidence supporting my pain. If you look for proof, you'll always find it online. The truth is, the folks who choose to take control of their painful situation, won't be found on the internet whining all day to anyone who'll listen. They're all out living life, instead of playing victim. What makes Emily's story intriguing is that she made such a strong association between her pain and cancer. Prior to her divorce, she hadn't known such physical discomfort, which only amplified her fear. That fear created more stress in her body, thus more pain. Imagine if another doctor told her that she had IBS or an ulcer- labels are documents of authenticity that people use as a crutch. Fortunately, this wasn't the case for Emily.

Here's some good news: *If you can dream up negative and destructive circumstances, you can also dream up positive and constructive alternatives.*

This next experiment doesn't require any writing (thanks a bunch, Rocco… sheesh… I just want to train people). Believe me; you'll thank me for this one. Instead of writing, this consists of field work. Whenever possible, get them sneakers on and maybe a warm coat (unless it's August). Do you have a "special place" that makes you feel at peace? Maybe when you were younger, you spent each summer at the lake. No? Fine, be that way- how about a beach that you enjoy walking on? If you don't have a favorite spot, create one. I love the beach at sunset. My wife and I end up there at least two or three times per week once the weather breaks. It doesn't matter what mood I'm in either, because the power of nature is far greater than whatever pettiness is going on inside me. Why picture a tranquil setting, when you can actually visit one?

Once you arrive at this place, start taking in all of your senses. What do you see around you? What sounds are in the distance? Perhaps there's a nostalgic aroma in the air. Feel the cool breeze pass through you as your journey begins.

Are you relaxed yet? Not yet? Move slowly through your path- there's no rush. If you're sitting, close your eyes for a moment and listen to your surroundings. If your mind is wandering, let it do so; don't try to force your thoughts out, but rather let them slip away naturally. All that matters is calmness. Your stresses have the rest of the day off- I've already sent them home.

What are your dreams? The sky's the limit, so think of your fondest desires. Don't be afraid- you can do anything here. No boundaries. No walls in front of you anymore. All that matters is you, nature and your dreams, all of which are connected. I'll do this part with you:

I dream of freedom. I want my wife and I to spend each day together, making music and watching the sunset. I don't want to work for someone anymore. I don't want to stand around helplessly, while she has to grind it out for us. I want us to live on this beach together. I want Sunday night to become the best time of the week, not the worst. I want us to be happy.

It's time to make your intentions clear. Your dreams are possible. They can happen for you. You deserve them as much as anyone else. Become the author of your destiny. Use words such as "I can" and "I shall." Command with passion your desires. I did and it was quite empowering:

> *My dreams are possible. I know I deserve the things I want. I am a resident of this world and claim my share of it's riches. I will have freedom. My life's work is here with my lady. I can bring my dreams into fruition and I will. I choose my life. This is my picture show. I'm in control of my story. I believe in my dreams. I believe in my dreams. I am grateful for this moment. I am grateful for having the potential to be here right now, doing this. Being unique is a good thing. I'm so proud of myself for choosing the narrow path, the path that most people are too afraid to walk on. My dreams are coming true. My dreams are coming true.*

> *Now simply relax and enjoy the moment. You won't soon forget it.*

I hope the last exercise inspired you. Inspiration is paramount to accomplishing your dreams and aiding in your clients dreams as well. I know that there are some who would suggest that you act as if you already have these dreams. For instance, by declaring "I can and will have my dreams," some think that by placing these affirmations in the future tense, will keep them there and never allow your dreams to exist in the present. That's simply untrue. In fact, doing the opposite (i.e. "I am wealthy" or "I live the life of dreams!"), can be discouraging. Take James, for example:

When I was twenty two, I had been working in a printing plant since high school ended. At first, like so many willing young men, I went to work excited at the chance to pull my own weight. That lasted maybe a few months, before I began to regret my decision to drop out of college. The work wasn't getting harder, but I was growing bored of the routine. I had also just moved in with my girlfriend, after she became pregnant. The bills were piling up, but our income was running scarce.

One morning, I pulled into my company parking lot and a friend came knocking on my window. He had heard some news and felt obligated to tell me first. They were letting me go. I was in shock. I worked my butt off for four years and never took sick time. Honestly, I don't remember asking my boss for anything in that time. Just the same, times were tough and other employees had seniority over me. I was able to go on unemployment for six months, but the payout was less than my old wages and we were already struggling. I spent the good part of a year searching for a job and finally found something in a warehouse. The pay wasn't good and the people had nasty attitudes. What could I do? My wife and newborn needed me.

After several months at the new job, I broke down. I became very depressed and felt ashamed of my position in life. I went to a therapist who had instructed me to decide what I want in life and live like I already have it. I told her that I wanted to be rich. Her response was "Then you must act as if you have the money now. Tell yourself that you are rich and have everything that you want. If you want a mansion, pretend that it's already bought." I took her advice and really got into it for a while. I drove around town acting as though I were Rockefeller. I didn't really believe it though. How could I lie to myself, when I was waking up to go to a degrading job every morning? I would say "I'm so rich, I am a multimillionaire," while my boss was cutting out our health benefits. I felt discouraged and out of despair, I found new ways of convincing myself that I was rich. I spent the little money we had on expensive flat screens and fancy restaurants. After all, rich people can easily do these things. Eventually, I couldn't take the rejection any longer and stopped going to therapy. I replaced it with my own model for success, one that worked for me. I knew that it was possible for anyone to become rich and I had always believed in myself. My altered affirmations went something like "I believe in myself and I believe that I will be rich. I will pursue my goals relentlessly until and I am determined to succeed."

It was hard at first, but I eventually overcame the obstacles and found a better job working with handicapped children. During that time, I had developed a business plan and opened a daycare center from home. My wife and son help run it and we live in total abundance, while helping others in the process.

It is important to note that James didn't let his temporary discouragement derail him from accomplishing his dreams. A simple shift in perspective, even replacing a few words, can make all of the difference. Although we can store any file in our unconscious facility, the strongest files are those that we believe in. If you live in a car (and I hope that isn't the case), telling yourself that you are wealthy is meaningless if you don't feel that way. Again, it's the feelings you put into your files that create the changes, not empty affirmations. If you tell yourself "I believe in myself and despite my situation, which is just a test, I will become rich," that may be more real for you than diluting yourself.

In contrast, I've studied people who possessed the amazing gift of believing they were the greatest champions of all time, while they were still learning how to box. In the case of Mohamed Ali, his forecast turned out to be true. His critics called him delusional and arrogant- yet, he inspired millions and gave so much of himself to children in need. Remember: It's what you

46

believe that counts the most. If you truly believe you are the richest man or woman alive, then go with that! If you honestly don't feel wealthy, create believable assertions that are still empowering for you. Here's a list of statements that can help you get into a healthier state of mind. Use the ones that make sense to you and scrap the rest. Type these up in 36 font size and tape 'em all over your home. Recite them often and *feel energized* as you do this! Here we go:

I Am In Control Of My Body And Mind!

I Can Do Everything That I Want!

I Deserve To Live In Abundance!

My Dreams Are Coming True!

I Am The Master Of My Life!

I Believe In My Dreams!

I Believe In Myself!

I Love Myself!

I Am Intelligent!

It's My Time To Shine!

I Have So Much To Offer!

I Am A Beautiful Human Being!

Making Millions Is Very Easy For Me!

I Will Fall In Love And Be Loved By A Great Person!

I Am Becoming A Successful Personal Trainer!

Take the cup above and drink it up! You may add to the glass or create additional ones. You can even arrange them into categories, if that suits you. The idea is to get you feeling good. Even though negative feelings may not have brought you to this book, it's the positive energy that makes the magic happen. Good work! Now go and relax- you're on your way to creating your own success as a trainer.

Exercise

Let's examine the basic fundamentals of exercise itself. What is exercise? On the surface, one mainstream definition is:

Any movement that requires physical and/or mental exertion especially
when performed to develop or maintain fitness.

Another common definition representing exercise:
A regular or repeated use of a faculty or bodily organ for the sake of enriching and maintaining physical fitness.

Although these definitions paint a picture of elementary focus, we need to illuminate a more detailed approach to the nuts and bolts of exercise. There are various dynamic elements that comprise of a typical workout. The main elements are:

1. Strength

2. Aerobic

3. Anaerobic
4. Balance

5. Coordination

6. Flexibility

7. Explosiveness

8. Cardiovascular
9. Endurance

10. Speed

11. Nutrition

12. Metabolism

13. Focus

14. Determination

Definitions

Strength: the utilization of one's optimum muscular force maximized by current physiological and/or psychological limitations.

Aerobic: physical movement that requires oxygen, which occurs during high volume, low intensity exercise.

Anaerobic: physical movement that works to increase muscle tissue without use of oxygen; occurring in high intensity, low volume exercise.

Balance: the state of equilibrium characterized by cancellation of equal opposing forces.

Coordination: the function of muscle groups in a

harmonious execution of movements.

Flexibility: the capability of withstanding stress without injury; adapting to physical or mental modification.

Explosiveness: a sudden and intense release of muscular energy, pulling and pushing in motion.

Cardiovascular: physical performance involving the heart and blood vessels, causing a temporary increase in heart rate.

Endurance: the physical and/or psychological capacity to bear hardship
or stress.

Speed: swiftness of action, measures the rate of motion.

Nutrition: food components that aid in nourishing the body, comprised of proteins, fats, carbohydrates, water, vitamins, and minerals.

Metabolism: the process in which nutrients enter the body and the rate at which they
are absorbed and utilized.

Focus: a center of activity or interest, in the state of optimal clarity or distinction.

Determination: firmness of resolution, the purposeful act of arriving at a decision.

Muscle Groups

As a qualified personal trainer, you will not be expected to memorize the entire human anatomy in order to fulfill client needs. Having said that, it is important to have a strong understanding of the major and minor muscle groups, the different body compositions, and of course, how each of them function.

To begin with, here are the main muscle groups in the

human body listed from head to toe:

Sterno Mastoids: the muscles located on each side of the neck, their function is to keep the head up and also rotate it.

Trapezius: these muscles are located behind the neck and begin the back muscles. Commonly referred to as the "Traps," they shrug the shoulders up and down.

Deltoids: these are the muscles that attach the arm to the shoulder joints and consist of the anterior (frontal), lateral (side) and posterior (back) deltoids. They are responsible for raising the arms to the sides and overhead.

Pectoralis Major and Minor: known as the "Pecs," they are the chest muscles that push weight away from the body.

Latissimus Dorsi: the muscles of the back that (when developed) look like the letter "V," respond to pulling objects from above or in a rowing motion. Also known as "Lats."

Biceps: located on the front of the arm, the biceps typically pull weight inward towards the body.

Triceps: located on the back of the arm, triceps push or straighten the arm outward, away from the body.

Forearm Muscles: responsible for turning the hand, the top of the forearm is called the *Brachialis* and the *Extensor Carpi* is on the lower forearm.

Rotator Cuff: this is actually made up of muscles in the upper back *also* involved in pulling weight inward and holds the arm and shoulder together. They are the *Rhomboids, Teres Major and Minor, Super-Spranatis, Infra-Spranatis,* and *Sub-Scapularis.*

Abdominals: the stomach muscles, which aid in core stabilization and offer relief to the lower back. The famous "Six Pack" phrase refers to these muscles.

Contrary to popular belief, the abdominal muscles work together as a unit, regardless of which area (upper/lower) is focused on. They contract in unison.

Obloquies: are found on the sides of the lower torso, they help twist the waist in all directions.

Spinal Erectors: also known as Lumbars, they are the lower back muscles that help us stand up straight after bending down.

Gluteus Maximus: the muscles of the buttocks, used to stand straight and extend the legs.

Quadriceps: the muscles of the upper legs, they aid in lifting objects from a squatting position as well as raising the knee.

Biceps Femorus: known as the "Hamstrings," these muscles stretch the heels upwards towards the buttocks or "Glutes." Some people have longer hamstrings than others, which explains why some are far more flexible than others (along with lower back problems or lack of stretching).

Gastrocnemeus: finally, the calf muscles behind the lower legs that help us jump and stand on our tiptoes.

Body Types

Human beings are made up of three different body types consisting of varying physiological characteristics. They are the *Endomorphs*, *Mesomorphs*, and *Ectomorphs*.

<u>Endomorphs</u> are generally characterized as having big bones, round faces, large thighs, and storage areas for body fat, usually around the waist. Weight control may be more challenging, though never impossible.

<u>Mesomorphs</u> tend to have a natural, lean looking body with fast metabolism. They typically need less exercise to gain muscle or lose weight compared to endomorphs. Their body structure is characterized by having broad shoulders, naturally larger muscles, thin waists, and faster metabolism.

Ectomorphs are known for having a thinner appearance. They often have smaller hips and shoulders. They also have a low body fat percentage. They are sometimes the "envied" group due to the fact that their metabolism provides them the benefit of eating more while remaining slim. The downside is that they lack in form or shape due to low muscle concentration.

A major point to understand is that there is no such thing as being 100% endomorph, mesomorph, or ectomorph. Everyone is made up of a combination of ALL three characteristics, though one body type usually dominates over the others.

Muscle Fiber

Depending on the specific training your client partakes in (i.e. weight lifting, aerobics, etc), there are three different fiber types, all present in each muscle. They are the fast twitch (*pennate*), medium twitch (*bi-pennate*) and slow twitch (*fusiform*). Fast twitch muscle fibers are correlated with regimens such as lifting heavy weight, football and martial arts. Notice all of these require explosive movement. During such performances, muscles will hypertrophy (grow) more than when medium or slow twitch fibers are utilized.

A good example of this is during a mass building routine. Let's say your client is bench pressing 70% of the maximum weight he/she can lift 1 time or rep. Doing so will optimize the fast twitch fiber response. Lifting heavier weight between 1-12 repetitions maximum, results in larger gains and is attributed to fast twitch muscle fibers. This is the most beneficial formula for building muscle mass.

It is useful to note medium twitch fibers (mainly because everyone has them), though most trainers focus primarily on fast and slow. The reason is that if someone wants to lose weight or prepare for a long distance marathon, the trainer will set up a routine that uses slow twitch muscle fibers. Their function is <u>not</u> to build muscle mass, but to aid in toning and endurance. As stated above, if a client wishes to build muscle, his/her trainer will emphasize the fast twitch muscle fibers. Medium twitch fibers work best during an exercise with repetitions between 12 and 20. Slow twitch fibers emanate best in repetitions over 25.

All three muscle fiber types automatically change from one to another depending on the actual routine. There is a strong connection between the muscle fiber functions and *volume* verses *intensity*.

Volume vs. Intensity Training

Similar to fast and slow twitch muscle fibers, another important method of determining the optimal regimen for a client is the *volume vs. intensity* model. The philosophy is simple:

Weight loss = high volume, low intensity exercise

Muscle building = high intensity, low volume exercise

High volume exercises include using the treadmill, light weight training with high repetitions, the stationary bike, abdominal work, and aerobics. High volume training is still the best known exercise method for burning calories and losing fat. The majority of women that will come to you will not be interested in building huge muscle mass. The key is to focus their weight loss routine on high volume, low intensity exercise. Using weight training is still important to help tone and maintain muscle development. If there is a lack of protein in their diet, when involved in a weight loss program, the human body needs energy to perform these exercises and will eventually tap into muscles for fuel. We will discuss basic nutrition later on. Keep in mind, when weight training in a high volume workout, make sure to use light weight and more repetition. It is also important to avoid using the stair master machines, because they are designed for higher intensity, lower volume workouts.

High intensity exercises include the bench press, using the stair climber, dead lifts, preacher curls, lat pull-downs, etc. Again, along with proper diet (the majority of ANY physical change in either weight gain or loss is the result of diet), quality mass building is best achieved by less repetitions, lifting heavier weights. This is in connection with fast twitch muscle fibers, though there are exceptions. For instance, if bodybuilders want to burn fat off of their stomachs, they may incorporate certain high volume abdominal exercises. This will give them a leaner look in that area, instead of turning 100% of the fat into muscle. But overall, high intensity, low volume exercise is paramount to gaining muscle mass.

Studies show the best muscle hypertrophy occurs during the last couple of reps; the last is known as a "forced rep." This is due to increased tearing of the muscles. There has been recent controversy on this subject and not all trainers agree on this, but many professional bodybuilders believe that in order to achieve *maximum* muscle growth, it is necessary to push to fatigue. In contrast, muscle gain does not need to result from pushing to complete failure each time. Honestly, this all depends on an individual's fitness goals. If they want to look like Arnold, perhaps pushing to fatigue will get them there faster. As a personal trainer, the most important piece of advice you will ever need to give someone is "train, don't strain." Safety should <u>always</u> come first.

Personal Training Tips: After a series of weight lifting exercises has been completed, your client may look more impressive than usual. This is referred to as the "pump." This literally means that blood has pumped into the muscles that have been training. Within a few hours, this look will fade. To insure they do not become discouraged (and blame it on their genetics), inform them that actual muscle growth occurs the days following the workout... NOT during. It is when they feel soreness that their muscles are rebuilding.

In a common weight loss situation, it is important for your client to be aware that calories are STILL burning off in the hour following their session. Because of this, it would be insurmountable to keep calories off if they eat a poorly constructed lunch right after. Though it is normal to grow hungry after a workout, proper nutrition is imperative.

Basic Nutrition

In this program, our emphasis is primarily on exercise and composition. Having said this, it is important as a personal trainer to understand the basics of proper and improper dietary habits. Your clients will undoubtedly seek advice on this subject as it goes hand in hand with exercise. Listed in this section is general dietary information that will assist you in your practice.

When asked about the value of proper nutrition, it may help to discuss the following main food sources: **Fat:** contains 9 calories per gram and has the most calories of all macronutrients. The "good" fats (or unsaturated fats) can be found in flaxseeds and fish oils. The "bad" (saturated and trans fats) are commonly found in red meat, bacon, dairy products, etc.

Calories: used in the measurement of nutritional energy properties. Typically in a weight loss diet, the rule of thumb is: the fewer the calories the better.

Cholesterol: a form of fat that is broken up into two main areas. HDL or "good" cholesterol is used to produce many hormones in the body. LDL or "bad" cholesterol builds up inside arteries and can lead to heart disease and stroke. Foods containing high levels of cholesterol are red meat, butter, egg yolks, etc.

Carbohydrates: In the past decade, there has been a major popularity boost in low carb diets (i.e. Ketogenic, Carnivore, Atkins, etc). Whereas it is better to avoid digesting too many grams of carbs for weight control, eating foods containing too few grams can be dangerous. For example, if switching to the Keto Diet, your body still needs carbs as a fuel source, at least while transitioning to fat as the primary source of energy (or Ketosis). Carbs are carbon, hydrogen and oxygen compounds that make up of sugars, starches and fibers. You can find them in pasta, certain candy, rice, etc. More on this subject in the Sports Nutritionist section.

Vitamins and Minerals: these are both organic and can be ingested. They are vital to life preservation and can be found in most foods. They support various bodily functions, including all systems.

Vitamin A: aids in growth, tissue repair, healthier skin, protection against disease and infection, eyesight, and external parasites. Found in eggs, liver, dairy products, cod liver oil, and supplements.

B Complex Vitamins: covers a wide range of functions including boosting energy, absorption of nutrients, nervous system optimization, lowering blood pressure, enhances heart functions, synthesis of amino acids, metabolism.

Vitamin C: ascorbic acid necessary for healing and protecting against disease, parasites, infection, anemia, nosebleeds, cavities, cancer, loss of appetite, joint pain, wounds. It can be taken as a supplement or found in citrus fruits and natural juices.

Vitamin D: main function is helping Calcium and Phosphorous absorption. It is also involved in stabilizing the nervous system and maintaining proper coronary function. Found in milk, soy, fish, orange juice, and cod liver oil.

Vitamin E: a fat-soluble vitamin essential for normal reproduction; an important antioxidant that neutralizes free radicals in the body. Antioxidants protect the cells of the body from the effects of free radicals, which have been known to cause cell damage which can contribute to the development of cardiovascular disease and cancer. Found in supplements, olive oil, egg yolks, and fish oils.

Magnesium: Magnesium is a mineral that is abundantly found in nature, and the human body contains about one ounce of magnesium, mostly in bones and muscles. It can found in both plant and animal sources, though plants provide a richer source. It may be one of the most important anti-aging minerals, and magnesium is essential for calcium and vitamin C absorption, as well as helping the metabolism of phosphorus, sodium, and potassium. It helps convert blood sugar into energy and it is necessary for effective nerve and muscle functioning. It is often referred to as the anti-stress mineral. Many people are deficient in this mineral because of reliance on processed foods and because magnesium is easily depleted by none other than stress.

Iron: helps the blood and muscles deliver oxygen to every body cell, and it removes carbon dioxide from them. It is important to immune system functions, and the body self-monitors and regulates the absorption and use of iron for varying needs. Benefits include a provision of energy, stronger immune system, and proper mental function. Found in liver, red meat, baked beans, pork, soy, black-eyed peas, fish, chicken, oatmeal, rye bread, whole wheat bread, and juices.

Potassium: the third most abundant mineral in the body and is considered an electrolyte. It can help to prevent high blood pressure and may enhance the effect of antihypertensive medications. Both physical and mental stress can lead to a deficiency in potassium. Alcohol, coffee, and sugar can deplete potassium levels. It is vital to maintaining a normal heartbeat or heart rhythm. Potassium also functions and enables the body to convert glucose into energy, which is stored in reserve by the muscles and liver.

Protein: the building blocks of muscle, protein is comprised of amino acids and is responsible for the growth and repair of muscle tissue. There are different forms of protein including animal and vegetable. One gram of protein contains four calories. For bodybuilders, it is important to consume enough protein to complement their intense workouts. On average, one gram of protein should be consumed daily for every pound of current body weight. Many people go even further by consuming one gram of protein for every desired pound of body weight. If your client's goal is to gain mass, this principle is helpful. There are so many people who become discouraged, because they do not realize the importance of eating while bulking up.

Selenium: a mineral that fights diseases such as cancer and heart disease. It is a potent antioxidant that helps slow down aging. It is essential to many body functions and can be found in all cells, but more so in the liver, kidneys, spleen, and pancreas.

Sodium: a mineral necessary for regulation of blood and body fluids, transmission of nerve impulses, heart activity, and certain metabolic functions. Most people consume excess amounts, usually in the form of table salt and can have a dangerous effect on the health.

Zinc: plays an important role in cell division, growth, and repair. It helps with healing and maintaining a sense of taste and smell. It can be useful in fighting colds, flu, and other infections. Zinc is a component of over 200 enzymes, most of which are involved in protein and DNA synthesis. It has beneficial effects on sex and thyroid hormones. Found in crab, red meat, turkey, ham, pork, chicken, eggs, seafood, beans, split peas, cereal, wheat germ, and brown rice.

Performance Supplements

Creatine: usually in powder form, helps maintain energy during a workout and faster recovery afterwards. Always follow directions on labels when using any supplement enhancer.

Protein Shake: they can play an important role for a person looking to gain muscle mass. There are many assortments of flavor, protein types (such as soy, egg, whey, and milk), brands, and quantities. Ask a health food store associate for information regarding proper selection.

Weight Loss Supplements: in all honesty, some of these do help stop food cravings and burn off weight… mostly water weight. BUT they are sometimes more dangerous to a person's overall health and should used with great care.

As with any worthy goal in life, self-discipline and hard work will always result in greater rewards. A magic pill cannot replace will power in the gym. All diet and exercise programs start within each individual, not from external sources. If someone you are training with uses any of the afore mentioned, suggest that they always take with caution.

Note:

Sufficient water intake is needed by the body throughout the day, especially after a good workout. It makes sense, being that 70% of our body is comprised of water. Individual organs raise that estimate even higher, such as the brain which is approximately 80% water. If your client is concerned about adding water weight, let them know it's not from water! Instead, suggest that they omit sugars, starches, soda, alcohol, and other high calorie food and beverages from their diet.

Assessment Tests

After the initial consultation with your new client, it is highly recommended that you issue a posture and flexibility assessment. This allows you to locate potential structural problems, such as rounding of the spinal cord that produces a "slouching" back posture look. When misalignment of the neck, back, shoulders, and hips occurs, not only will it become more difficult to train your client, but it can also lead to health related problems later on. To perform these tests on anyone should be simple and gentle, yet the benefits of doing so will be rewarding. Just being consciously aware of these areas can help them to improve dramatically. As always, write down all information in your journal and suggest he/she does the same.

Proper head posture will result from practicing keeping the head held straight up over the shoulders. When the head is misaligned, the chin usually looks pushed forward, creating a lazy neck position.

To adjust head and upper back posture, have your client stand up straight in their usual position. From a side angle, again, notice the afore mentioned chin position and see if their shoulders look rounded or slumped forward. If this is the case, it is due to weak muscles in the upper back as well as tightening of the chest and shoulders.

For the lower back, again from the side angle, see if the head and shoulders align straight with the hips and ankles. Your client should look slightly curved around the neck and above the buttocks. This is normal. If the lower back looks too arched or concaved, the muscles of the lower back are doing too much work. In contrast, if their lower back is convex or at least flattened, you may notice bent knees.

Abdominal and hip flexor work will help, because they can take some of the work load off the back safely. Remind them that the stomach should never stick out past the chest. Much of the time, people will see that as having a lot of fat in the stomach, but this is not always the case. Proper posturing along with core training can help solve this.

Quality stretching methods include:

Neck: you can have them slowly roll their neck in a circular motion and change directions after several seconds. They can also slowly lift their head to the ceiling, hold for a second, then slowly bring it down so the chin can tuck naturally over the chest.

Arms: the first stretch is simply to have them straighten each arm out to the side and make wide circles in one direction. After about 8-10 seconds, change direction. Once both arms have been stretched individually, they can circle both together. The second arm stretch involves both hands interlocking at the fingers and stretching both palms outward, so that both arms are at chest level. Hold for five seconds and release.

Shoulders: standing up straight with hands at both sides, ask them to turn their palm facing behind their lower back. They will then raise their hand up towards the opposite shoulder blade. If they cannot reach it, "practice makes *better*." They can also perform this from behind their head as well. Another good stretch is to lock both hands together behind the back and lift up the arms slowly.

Lower Back: have your client lie down on his/her back and use both hands to draw in both knees towards their chest (pulling behind the thighs is easier). If they can touch their chest with their knees, they probably have good flexibility in the lower back. The popular "Cat Stretch" also works well. To do this, have them sit with their buttocks down on the heels of the feet in an upright position. They then raise both hands stretched above their head and slowly lower the arms and upper body outward and down toward the floor. From there, they can slowly glide their chest forward and end up in a modified push-up position, with both arms locked and holding up the torso, while the head looks up at the ceiling.

Buttocks: from standing position, have them pull one knee up with both hands towards their chest. Hold for five seconds, then release the knee slowly and perform the same stretch with the other knee.

Thighs: from standing position, have them lift one foot behind the body and grab with same side hand. The key to balance, is to focus the eyes on one spot in front of them. They can also lay down on their stomach, legs straight and knees together. Have them draw one heel in towards the buttocks and hold it there with the same side hand.

Hamstrings: from standing position, feet no more than shoulder widths apart, ask them to bend their body down towards the floor without bending the knees. See if they can reach the ground with their outstretched hands. Next, have them lie on the ground (on their back) and slowly raise one leg upward without bending the knee. Arms remain at both sides during full exertion.

Calves: have them sit on the ground in an upright position (they can use their arms to support them by leaning back on them slightly). With their legs out straight in front of them, they then pull their toes back towards their shins and hold them upward for no more than five seconds before pointing them outward again. Make sure they do not lift their heels off the floor. Another good calf stretch is performed in the standing position and have them slowly lift up on to the balls of their feet and slowly back down again while keeping the legs straight.

Testing their posture in motion will also help them to recover proper posture while everyday walking. There are easy methods of testing this. The first, is to simply have them walk in their normal fashion 10-15 paces (not on a plank) back and forth while you check their alignment. Another way is to use a step platform, no more than six inches in height, have them step up onto it one foot at a time repeatedly. It should look as if they are walking up stairs in place.

You may use any of these exercises before the main training section begins. Try to be consistent by starting at the neck and working your way down to the feet. Always remember: "You rush it, you ruin it." Try to make sure they move through all stretches slowly. They will have plenty of time during each workout to pick up the pace. Though
it is always a safe bet to go through these stretches with each client, ask that they begin warm-ups before the session, so stretching doesn't take too much time.

Heart Rate

There are two ways of measuring heart rate. You can use a heart rate monitor, which will give you fast and precise results. These days, you can wear a monitor on your wrist (like a watch) and easily check it at any time. Always keep track of battery power, so your client doesn't freak out if there is no pulse reading.

If you want to wait on using a monitor, you can also use your finger tips and press on your client's radial artery on the wrist. Make sure you <u>never</u> use their neck to check pulse count. During their exercise session, it is helpful to gage their heart rate by placing your index and middle fingers on their wrist and once you have found their pulse, count 10 full beats. Make sure you start counting their heart beats right after they stop the activity; you will only have a 15 second window of accuracy. Once you have obtained their 10 second pulse, multiply that number by 6. This determines their heart rate in beats per minute or BPM.

Age	Target Heart Rate During Exercise
18-30	98-146 beats per minute

31-40	93-138 beats per minute
41-50	88-131 beats per minute
51-60	83-124 beats per minute
61+	78-116 beats per minute

Exercise Routine

To begin with, it is recommended that you explain certain terms with your client before your training session starts. For instance, a *repetition* or rep, is the number of times they will lift and lower weight in the course of one set. A *set* is a series made up of reps. In between sets, is the rest period. One minute of rest should be sufficient. If they need more time, that is acceptable, but keeping their heart rate and muscles stimulated is how good results are achieved.

Training With Weight (Isotonic Training)

In your experience as a trainer, you will find that there is no shortage of weight training theories. In this section, we will cover the standard and <u>safe</u> method of training. Remember, a personal trainer has many responsibilities and safety is ranked number one.

When first starting, a client may only wish or financially be able to train with you once per week. If this is so, explain to them that for optimum results, they should train at least three times per week depending on their specific goals.

If you are only able to train your client once per week, try to include at least 8-10 exercises that cover the major muscle groups. Normally, it helps to train each muscle group twice per week (on alternate days), but studies show that working each group even once per week can be quite effective. There are plenty of exercises to choose from when building size or toning up. If they are looking to add mass, they should use weight that they can only lift 6-12 reps with good form. If they are interested in losing weight or toning, they should use light weight and perform at least 12-25 reps per set. There is no golden rule for the amount of sets per exercise. In the beginning, try one set per exercise and even one exercise per muscle group. For losing weight, you can also have your client perform <u>certain</u> exercises with the goal of reaching 100 reps straight. Naturally, such training (referred to as *circuit training*) should always be performed using very light or no weight and must be built up over time. It is important to explain to them that though diet is the key component to weight loss, exercise and nutrition balance well together. Here is a sample list and instructions for each exercise:

<u>**Chest**</u>

Barbell Bench Press: have your client lie on his/her back on a bench, with feet firmly rooted on the floor in front. Gripping the bar firmly with both hands (broader than shoulder width), have them slowly lower the weight down to the center of
their chest and slowly raise it back up. Make sure they keep their hips on the bench at all times.

Dumbbell Bench Press: have your client lie on his/her

back on a bench, with feet firmly rooted on the floor in front. Holding a dumbbell in each hand, have them start by bringing the dumbbells at about shoulder level, close to their body and palms facing their feet. They then push the weights out until their arms are straight and over their chest (not the head). Slowly lower the weights down again. Make sure they don't lift their head during motion.

Incline Dumbbell Press: follow the same guidelines as stated above, only this time the actual bench back has been elevated to work the upper pecs. Make sure the bench isn't elevated to steep of an angle.

Dumbbell Flyes: have your client lie on their back on a bench, holding dumbbells in each hand. Next, they should hold both arms out over their chest, palms facing each other. With elbows bent, they slowly bring the weights out and down to their sides, so they are parallel with the bench. Lastly, slowly raise the weights back up. Make sure their arms don't go down too low!

Elastic Band Press: using elastic resistance cables or

bands (attached to a wall or using a door strap), have your client hold a band in each hand and in a standing position, facing away from the wall, slowly push out the bands until arms are straightened. This should be a wide angle, broader than shoulder width to maintain full range of motion. Slowly return bands to starting position.

Shoulders

Seated Dumbbell Press: ask your client to sit on the end of a bench, keeping both feet grounded in front. holding a dumbbell in each hand, press the weight in a steady motion up and overhead so they nearly touch each other, keeping elbow slightly bent at the top. Slowly lower the weight to starting position. Make sure they keep their palms facing in front during full motion and have them look directly in front at all times.

Front Dumbbell Raise: standing up, with feet shoulder width apart, have your client slowly raise one arm straight out in front, until the weight is just above shoulder height. As they lower the weight, their other arm should begin the same motion. This is excellent for the anterior deltoids. Make sure they do not lean or sway forward or backwards during this exercise.

Side Dumbbell Raise: standing up, with feet shoulder width apart, have your client slowly raise one arm out to their side, until the weight is just above shoulder height. As they lower the weight, their other arm should begin the same
motion. This is excellent for the lateral deltoids. Make sure they do not lean or sway forward or backwards during this exercise.

Shoulder Shrugs: standing up, with feet shoulder width apart and holding a dumbbell in each hand at their sides, have your client slowly lift their shoulders up, while keeping their arms down at their sides. Slowly lower shoulder. This is especially good for the traps.

Biceps

Seated Dumbbell Curls: have your client sit on the end of a bench in an upright position, while holding a dumbbell in each hand. Keeping elbows at their sides, they will slowly curl their arms up towards their shoulders, either one at a time or together. Slowly lower weight. Make sure they don't sway or lean backwards.

Standing Barbell Curls: standing up, with feet shoulder width apart and holding a bar with both hands (shoulder width grip), the bar should be just in front of their thighs, palms facing out. Keeping elbows at their sides, have them slowly raise the bar until it stops just above their chest. Make sure they don't lean back.

Hammer Curls: standing up, with feet shoulder width apart and holding a dumbbell in each hand at their sides (palms facing sides), have them slowly raise their forearms up towards their shoulders, keeping upper arms and torso stationary. Slowly lower weight. This is also useful for training the forearms.

Triceps

Bench Dips: have your client stand with their back to a bench or even a chair. As they bend their legs, they will place their hands behind them on the edge on the bench, feet in front so weight is resting on arms. Slowly bend arms (elbows at sides), until upper arms are even with the floor. Their buttocks should end up inches from the floor. Slowly straighten arms to starting position. Make sure they don't lower their body too much.

Lying Dumbbell Extensions: have your client lie on their back on a bench, holding dumbbells in each hand. Next, they should hold both arms out in front of their head, palms facing each other. Bending their elbows, they should slowly lower the weight towards their shoulders, without moving their upper arms. The key is to have the elbows pointing upwards at the point of extension. Slowly return to starting position. Make sure they keep the elbows in (not outward) and don't aim weight near their head at any point.

<u>**Back**</u>

One Arm Dumbbell Row: have your client place their left knee on a bench, with their right foot on the floor. They will then bend their upper body forward so it is parallel to the bench. Use their left hand on the bench to support their weight, as

the right hand is holding a dumbbell straight down towards the floor. Looking straight ahead, have them pull their right elbow back as far as possible, without straining. Slowly lower weight. Make sure they keep their back flat and not rounded.

Wide Grip Pull-Down: have your client sit on a pull-down machine and adjust the knee pads so it fits comfortably. Gripping the bar above shoulder width apart, have them slowly lower the bar until it reaches in front of their collarbone. Make sure they don't lower it too far. Slowly raise the bar back up.

Legs

Dumbbell Squats: standing up, with feet shoulder width apart and holding a dumbbell in each hand at their sides, palms facing in, have them bend their legs at the knees and lower their hips until their thighs are parallel to the floor. Slowly use their legs to stand up. Make sure they always keep their back straightened and use only their legs during motion. This is great for the quadriceps!

Dumbbell Lunges: standing up, with feet shoulder width apart and holding a dumbbell in each hand at their sides, have them step forward with their right foot. While bending their knees, their hips should be lowered until the left knee is inches away from the floor. They then push their right leg up into standing position. Make sure their right knee bends just over the foot, but not too far over. When performed correctly, this is a tremendous quad exercise.

Angled Calf Raise: standing up, with feet shoulder

width apart and holding a dumbbell in each hand at their sides, have them turn their toes outward a couple of inches. They should then stand up on their toes, while keeping their arms at their sides. Slowly lower feet to starting position.

Abdominals

Floor/Ball Crunches: ask your client to lie on his/her back on a mat/ball. Have them place their hands beside their head just touching their ears. Drawing their knees up with feet flat on the floor, they should press their lower back down, while slowly bringing their shoulders up only 4-6 inches off the ground. Slowly return shoulders down, still concentrating on pushing their lower back into the floor/ball. Make sure they do not lock their hands behind their neck.

Twist Crunches: ask your client to lie on his/her back on a mat. Have them place their hands beside their head just touching their ears. Drawing their knees up with feet flat on the floor, let their knees fall over to one side as far as possible. They should press their lower back down, while slowly bringing their shoulders up only 4-6 inches off the ground. The focus here is on their obliques. Slowly return shoulders down, still concentrating on pushing their lower back into the floor and switch leg position. Make sure they do not lock their hands behind their neck.

Bent Knee Raises: ask your client to lie on his/her back on a mat. Have them place their hands beside their head just touching their ears. Drawing their knees up with feet flat on the floor, they should place a <u>light</u> dumbbell between both feet and slowly lift their knees up towards their chest. Make sure they keep their back flat and don't use heavy weight. Slowly lower the knees to the floor.

Treadmill: the use of a treadmill is a great way to burn off calories. Since this can take up training time, use it as a warm up for the first five minutes if weight loss is the desired goal. They also help increase heart rate and provides an exceptional method for warming up.

Note on Breathing: *during all exercises, full and steady breathing should be practiced. Remind them to inhale slowly during contraction and exhale during release. This may take time for some to adjust, but correct breathing is a fundamental habit to form.*

Helpful Tips

The average percentage of body fat for men is 8-12% and 12-16% for women. The easiest way to measure is by: Under the skin is a layer of fat and the percentage of total body fat can be measured by using the thumb and the index finger and pick up the skinfold at selected points on the body and then apply a pair of calipers. Ensure that all of the skinfold measurements are located on the right side of the body and that the measurements are taken in millimeters (follow caliper instructions before applying to anyone!). You can also buy electronic devices that are accurate and easy to use.

Of all attributes a personal trainer must possess, there is none more important than his/her ability to listen, inquire, and observe. Remember, you are not helping your clients to reach *your* goals. Something brought them to you. Even if they are not concise as to their specific needs or seem a bit cloudy when conveying them, make sure to hear what they are saying, especially during the initial consultation. Some people will be insecure and thus apprehensive in sharing their feelings with a stranger. That is not to say you should assume anything (what does assuming make?). You will learn that there are usually deep rooted reasons why so many people come to a trainer for help, deeper than merely looking good on a beach. Whereas you are not a doctor or psychologist and are not qualified to offer diagnosis, being a good listener goes a long way.

When discussing their health history, it is imperative for a trainer to become fully aware of any challenges that may result in injury. Each potential client has a unique situation. One woman might be getting ready for an upcoming police test. The demands of a physical agility exam can be stressful. If she needs to perform 20 push-ups, 30 sit-ups, and run 1.5 miles all in under 14 minutes, then these are the areas in which you must focus on. She may have the amazing ability to curl 60 lb dumbbells and build biceps well. Working her strong point is important, but remember the goals she came to you with in the first place.

Conversely, if a man with a history of lower back pain comes to you with a desire to become a professional body builder, you may need to stress the importance of core stability, focusing on abdominal strength (this can help take the load off of hip flexors and the lower back). Naturally, a big part of your job is encouragement, but always keep safety first and use my motto:

"Train, don't strain."

Asking questions is also a vital part of being a fitness trainer. After all, you are more of a personal guide than anything... but you are also a professional. Asking necessary questions will challenge your client to assess themselves in ways they could not have thought of on their own. There may also be occasions when a client is training and begins to feel dizzy or fatigued, but is afraid of quitting. Some might see this as an act of personal failure and may choose to keep quiet and continue. Pay attention to body language and ask how they are feeling throughout the workout.

As in the example above, not only will you help prevent injury by asking basic questions, but being a good observer goes hand in hand with listening, inquiring, and verbal communication. Sometimes, a faint look of boredom or heavy breathing is more than enough to promote questions. If a client say's "I'm fine, I'm fine," but is curled up in the fetal position, good observation skills can aid in avoiding such incidents.

Though these pointers are the most valuable tools in your new toolbox, the only way you will truly sharpen them is through real experience. Be patient with yourself. It takes time to master any worthy skill, but once you do, your life and the lives of your clients will grow into great fruition. You will spend a large amount of time keeping them from discouragement. Remember the saying "Practice what you preach."

Aerobics

Many companies offer separate aerobics certification programs and can be of great value to you as a fitness professional. If you are not interested in pursuing this added certification, as a personal trainer, you *still* need to understand the most popular form of exercising in the world.

Aerobic literally means "with <u>oxygen</u>" and includes any type of exercise, usually performed at lower to moderate intensity levels. Oxygen helps to burn fat and glucose in order to produce *Adenosine Triphosphate*, the main energy carrier for all <u>cells</u>. Some popular types of aerobic exercises include:

Running

Martial Arts/Qigong

Kickboxing Aerobics

Step Aerobics

CrossFit (will be discussed further later)

Advanced Pilates

Power walking

Swimming

Bicycling

Aerobic dancing

Skiing

Ice skating

Racket Ball

Rowing

The benefits of any aerobics program are: More stamina, weight loss, muscle tone increase, more energy, better sleep patterns, improved moods, healthier heart function, and elevated self-confidence.

The following guidelines will enable you to structure your beginner classes in a proficient and safe manner. Try to implement a minimum of 8 - 10 exercises, involving all major muscle groups, 2 times per week. 1 set of 8 - 12 repetitions of each exercise is recommended at first. Have your clients wear sneakers and light weight, well "breathing" clothing.

Another way to motivate clients is the use of music in an aerobics class. Play music that is upbeat (100-150 beats per minute or BPM) during peak periods and slower music during warm up and cool down sections. Obviously, try not to select anything offensive, but make it something contemporary (though the occasional 70's disco can make someone's day).

Aerobics classes are usually made up of 10 minute of warm-ups, 30 minutes of dance/step aerobics and a 5 minute cool down period. Use can eventually introduce light weight dumbbells and weighted ankle wraps to your program. Make sure to use no more than 2 lb. weights and spread everyone apart to avoid injury.

Low-Impact Aerobics: this is characterized as aerobic movements where at least one foot touches the ground at all times. This helps prevent leg, back and knee injuries and is useful for beginners, senior citizens and women who are pregnant.

High-Impact Aerobics: aerobic movements (such as jumping) where both feet come off the ground. The cardiovascular benefits increase with high-impact regimens, but make certain each client is physically prepared before they engage.

Step Aerobics: aerobics routine utilizing stepping up and down from a raised surface (stairs, stepper, Bosu). This is generally low-impact, but can be a high intensity work out. Always maintain proper form and balance throughout each movement.

Your First Session

Again, there are separate certifications for aerobics instructors to attain, but this basic information will be of enormous use (i.e. working with clients looking to lose weight and tone up). During a basic warm up section of your aerobic routine (post stretching phase), have your clients march in place, exaggerating their arms and legs. Next, you can demonstrate frontal heel to toe steps (step one heel out in front and back on the heel in rhythm with the music). Simultaneously, have them reach their arms out in front, bring them back and then up overhead and return down. You can develop your own hand and foot patterns (i.e. switch to squatting and reaching down and back up again). After they complete 20 reps, counting up to 10 and back down to 0, shift into front lunges. Have them push out their arms in various directions. After 20 reps, introduce side steps where they will step to their side with one foot and follow it with the other, then back again. Finally, have clients shift their weight on one leg and reach up with the opposite hand, then switch to the opposite leg. Repeat for 15-20 reps.

The pace of the music can pick up now, signifying higher intensity. While marching in place, the power arm punches straight out <u>while</u> the hips turn with it. The back foot also pivots out. This is where the true power comes form. After impact, the arm retracts rapidly back into guard position and the opposite arm repeats. The punch should snap out. They should always keep the knees slightly bent, so their legs don't lock up. 20 reps are sufficient during most of these exercises. Next, demonstrate *arm scissors,* by literally crossing both hands in a scissors fashion, while still marching in rhythm. You can implement creative step aerobics like used for warming up, only now it's faster and you can even add a stepper or Bosu (while they march in place, one foot steps up on the stepper/Bosu, comes back down while the other foot comes up).

Next, employ knee variations: While marching, lift either knee into high chamber position straight up while contracting abdominal muscles. For a curved knee, pivot front foot out and turn hips with it. Then, return to fighting stance. Use arms as a "goal post" to swing through the knee strike. Always return arms to guard position. Move into front kicks: Raising either knee one at a time, kick same leg out in front in a snapping motion. Curl toes back so that the ball of the foot makes contact. Return back to high knee (or chamber) position and down again. Keep feet light during all kicks. Do not try to muscle power out of their legs. Now, they are ready to merge the punches with the kicks. Use basic combinations such as a left cross punch, followed by a right front kick and so on. Once they are advanced, try adding 1-2 lb. dumbbells or wrist wraps to the session. Finally, there is no better way to end a high paced workout than with jumping jacks! By this point in the routine, their limbs should feel bricks- so a simple exercise will burn the most.

During the cool down phase, your clients can march in place and then have them follow you around in a circle while jogging. You can finish the routine with some push-ups, crunches or simple stretches. You can also work the abs with an exercise ball or Bosu. To execute a crunch from the ball, have them lie on their backs on a mat/ball. Have them place their hands beside their head just touching their ears. Drawing their knees up with feet flat on the floor, they should press their lower back down, while slowly bringing their shoulders up only 4-6 inches off the ground. Slowly return shoulders down, still concentrating on pushing their lower back into the floor/ball. Make sure they do not lock their hands behind their neck. To focus on their obliques, have them perform a crunch, only this time they will turn their elbows up and over towards the opposite side. Always let them know how good they did, so they'll keep attending classes.

At first, each client should have no more than 3 aerobics classes per week. It is perfectly normal to gradually build up one at a time. Remember, safety <u>always</u> comes first.

Enroll in an aerobics class. It is necessary to lead by example in this business, so make sure you are in decent shape and can handle the workouts you expect your clients to do.

Note: *if someone becomes fatigued or dizzy, have them stop exercising and walk with you slowly out of class range. Sit them down and give them water. Help them find their breath, because* *they are suffering from lack of oxygen to the brain. They should also stop for the day.*

TIP: *in a common weight loss situation, it is important for your client to be aware that calories are STILL burning off in the hour following their session. Because of this, it would be insurmountable to keep calories off if they eat a poorly constructed lunch right after. Though it is normal to grow hungry after a workout, proper nutrition is imperative.*

CASE STUDIES

Case Study One:

When "Kristina" first came to me for personal training, I sat with her and discussed the Health Questionnaire she had filled out, along with the Personal Training Goals, and release forms. Her goal was to lose twenty pounds, but she was concerned that she'd have to omit eating to do so. I explained to her that not only would "starving" herself be unnecessary, but in fact, it would also be counterproductive. The body needs proper nourishments to function correctly, *especially* when embarking on a new training regimen. During exercise, when the body is lacking in the right nutrients, it will need to tap into muscles as an energy source.

She smiled in relief as I continued to map out a daily diet that would correlate with her new training curriculum. In order to maintain a body fat percentage between 12-16 percent, we needed to cut down on calories found in a lot of junk foods, soda, milk, cake, and breads. Obviously, foods high in fat like French fries and bacon were taken out. A great importance in breakfast was mentioned. She was not looking to Hulk out and get ripped, so I made her aware of the amount of protein she had been consuming- she couldn't lose twenty pounds, if she took in as much protein as a pro body builder. I suggested she cut out the late night snacks, because it'll pretty much sit in her stomach all night, while nothing is being done to burn it off. For breakfast, I recommended using egg beaters and make an omelet with mixed fruit. Since she couldn't stay away from cheese, I enlightened her on the miracle of soy (though too much soy can be binding.) For lunch, a tossed salad with rice chopped up chicken breasts would go nicely with grape juice. For dinner, she could change it up with fish and celery sticks. If cholesterol is a factor, she might add carrots to her meals. Plain popcorn is a terrific snack; a small sandwich bad is good to determine proper portions. Since we're all different, I monitored her progression each week. If she lost too many calories, we added hot green tea to her breakfast.

For her training, I recommended she see me three times per week. Eventually, when ready, she may add a home routine. I expressed that since this is a big change for her, we shouldn't jump in too fast. I gave her a daily journal to write in during all workouts, as well as goal/progress sheets. During the first week, she was able to do about twenty-forty squats, front and side leg raises, lunges, and about fifteen crunches. We always stretched before these routines. She understood that a high volume workout was best for her goals, but got bored of the same exercises… NO problem!

By the third week, she was up to a hundred light dumbbell raises, calf raises, and rowing reps. We focused more on her lower body and saw results quickly. She hadn't realized that ALL of her abs were getting trained together, except her obloquies, which we used a ball for. She began using a stationary bike at home, but continued working with me. I saw a positive change in both her attitude and weight, which flattered me. I gained good referrals out of it as well.

Case Study Two:

After assessing all of "Herman's" paperwork, I learned that he had tried to lift weights and build muscle mass once before to no avail. I informed him that most problems young men have in gaining mass stem from their diet. Though it is probable he never had a motivator like me before and his weight lifting routine wasn't up to par, I could see his frustration after working hard in the gym mainly revealed his lack of protein each day. He was surprised when I told him he really should eat one gram of protein for every pound of body weight. "This doesn't mean you should run over to Taco Hell and order the whole menu, then dead lift the restaurant six times and go sleepies with the franchise in your system for three days."

For breakfast, drink a big glass of water or O.J., cook about a dozen egg whites, toast a plain bagel, and take a multi-vitamin. Within three hours, take a protein shake, and possibly throw in a banana. For lunch, eat an 8oz steak, veggies, a couple of baked potatoes, and add three amino acids. Later, before dinner, add another shake. Theoretically, dinner should be about the same as lunch. A substitution of chicken or fish, with a small portion of pasta is O.K. For desert, try half the amount of egg whites consumed for breakfast. Eventually, I introduced Creatine to his regimen. Besides spending more money in the grocery store, he was pretty happy.

Since he wished to build more muscle, I trained him using a high intensity work out. We started slowly, then had him pushing forced reps. I told him that as hard as it is to knock out the last two or three reps in an exercise, those were the ones that counted the most. It really helped him to carry his daily journal to each workout. It kept him disciplined and showed his progress. At first, it was tough for him to see the results in the mirror, but the journal was testimony. We worked each muscle once per week and trained in a four-day split. That motivated him and helped pay our phone bill at home. On Monday's and Wednesday's, we worked his legs, shoulders, abs. Tuesday's and Thursday's we did chest, arms, and a bit of self-defense… he was getting picked on by a four foot Asian girl from the office. We switched exercises between bench pressing, crunches, flies, inclined bench, lat pull downs, dumbbell curls, front dumbbell raises, dips, leg curls, squats, and shrugs with heavy weight five to eight sets of six to twelve to reps.

It didn't take too long before he achieved his goal. He understood that in order to maintain his physique, he had to stay on his program, gradually increasing weight as needed. Soon, all of the girls in the office stopped beating him up and asked him out instead. I was happy and so was he.

Case Study Three:

"Franklin" is a teacher in an elementary school and spends most of his day either standing at the black board or sitting at his desk. I wanted to get a good feel of how well he would adjust to a new diet and exercise routine. Without boring or confusing him, I explained the idea of a slow twitch muscle fiber type of program and healthier diet. Realizing his body fat is pushing 30 percent, I had to be cautious in my approach. He didn't seem too motivated and his self-esteem was under the floor boards. I also sensed skepticism, so I wanted to gain his trust first. We spoke between visits about different areas of interest. He, like me, loved watching horror flicks. That started us off on the right foot.

I casually mentioned the appropriateness of working a three day per week system, but he was reluctant at first. I was able to get him in once a week for a while, then twice, until he felt more comfortable and positive. Once he got used to the work outs and dietary changes, I worked with him three days per week. Similar to "Kristina's" nutritional scale, I put "Franklin" on a low fat diet. He was pretty lazy at first and I didn't want to chase him away, so we agreed that he would follow this routine ONLY on the days we would meet. For breakfast, I recommended using egg whites and make an omelet with mixed fruit. Since he couldn't stay away from bacon at first, I instructed him on turkey bacon. Eventually (once he couldn't stand turkey bacon any longer), he stopped bacon completely. For lunch, a tossed salad was out of the question for him, so chicken breasts with corn and apple juice would do. For dinner, he didn't mind fish and broccoli. Since cholesterol was a factor, he cut out the beer during watching Wrestling. No-fat pretzels and flavored water were O.K. as a replacement. Being weary of his fragile mental state, I let him know that "We all slip up on our diets now and then. Don't kick yourself too much when it happens, tell me instead and we'll figure it out." He loved that!

On alternating days, he worked up to three sets of twenty crunches and leg raises. To change it up, we used the ball on occasion. He did three sets of eight leg extensions and leg curls. Lunges were great, but they usually made him very sore for days after, so I suggested hot-tubs and massages, which he made no trouble about. He did three sets of eight lat pull downs and cable rows and the same for bench presses and machine presses. Naturally, we rotated each of these exercises by the day. Triceps presses and dumbbell kickbacks were also completed at three sets of eight. If he struggled, we stopped and took a breather. I tried to keep him from resting past a minute, but he loved to talk, so I slowly got him back on the weights while finishing up our conversations. We always started and ended our work outs with abs. It kept them stimulated that way, but I never over worked him.

My motto after working with "Franklin" became "Train, don't strain." In the end, he continued working with me and made full time changes to him diet. Not only was he looking great, but his attitude improved two hundred percent.

Conclusion

By this point, you have learned the

fundamentals a personal trainer should possess upon entering this ever-growing field. Continue to use this manual as a reference when needed and always look to increase your range of expertise. You will come to know great rewards as a role model and inspirational figure. That's a lot to be proud of, especially in a time of great global challenge. If you can help improve the life of just one person, your character will inherit the strength of a hundred. When embarking on any new venture, there will be times of worry and doubt. Always remember:

A person who walks with integrity will always have a road beneath their feet.

CHAPTER TWO:

SPORTS NUTRITION CONSULTANT

Nutrition

Nutrition is the process of nourishing or being nourished by which an organism assimilates food and uses it for:

If each of us needs to consume such nutrients, what are some of the different nutrients we use, what are they made up of and how do we process them? In this section, you will learn the mechanics of food sources in our bodies and different dietary approaches. This information has been designed to add quality to your new business. Feel free to print out any terms or theories and refer back to them as needed.

Macronutrients

Macronutrients are the nutrients that together provide the majority of metabolic energy to an organism. The three main macronutrients are proteins, carbohydrates, and fats. Other macronutrients include alcohol and organic acids. They are distinguished from Micronutrients (vitamins and minerals) because they provide energy to the body.

Protein: comes from the Greek Protas meaning "of

primary importance" and is a complex, high-molecular-mass, organic compound comprised of amino acids. They are essential to the structure and function of all living cells in the body. Different proteins perform a variety of functions. Certain proteins are enzymes, which catalyze chemical reactions. Other proteins help form the joints of the skeleton, while others build muscle tissue. Proteins make up specific sequences of amino acids. The details of these sequences are stored in the codes of all human genes. Proteins work together to achieve a particular function and associate with one another to form a complex (or group). Different proteins come from dairy, whey, egg, meat, and soy.

Carbohydrates: they are carbon, hydrogen and oxygen compounds that make up of sugars, starches and fibers. Your body needs them as a fuel source. Carbs are important storage and transport vessels of energy in most organisms, mainly plants and animals. They are categorized by their number of sugar units: monosaccharides (glucose and fructose), disaccharides (sucrose and lactose), oligosaccharides, and polysaccharides (starch, glycogen, and cellulose). You can find them in pasta, potatoes, candy, rice, etc. Fats: contains 9 calories per gram and has the most calories of all macronutrients. The "good" fats (or unsaturated fats) can be found in flaxseeds and fish oils. The "bad" (saturated and trans fats) are commonly found in red meat, bacon, dairy products, etc. Avoiding fast foods can be the most beneficial piece of advice you can give someone!

***Calories: used in the measurement of nutritional energy properties. Typically in a weight loss diet, the rule of thumb is: the fewer the calories the better. The average 2 liter bottle of soda contains 200 calories per serving!

*** *Calories are not considered macronutrients or micronutrients, but are used in measuring food properties.*

Micronutrients

Vitamins, minerals, antioxidants, and phytochemicals are considered Micronutrients because, in comparison with Macronutrients, they are needed by the body in smaller amounts. Our bodies need them to extrapolate energy out of carbs and fats and transform our protein consumption into muscle mass. They aid in the fight against cancer, AIDS, stroke, and also free radicals.

Vitamins and Minerals: these are both organic and can be ingested. They are vital to life preservation and can be found in most foods. They support various bodily functions, including all systems.

Vitamin A: aids in growth, tissue repair, healthier skin, protection against disease and infection, eyesight, and external parasites. Found in eggs, liver, dairy products, cod liver oil (yummy), and supplements.

B Complex Vitamins: covers a wide range of functions including boosting energy, absorption of nutrients, nervous system optimization, lowering blood pressure, enhances heart functions, synthesis of amino acids, and benefit metabolism.

Vitamin C: ascorbic acid necessary for healing and protecting against disease, parasites, infection, anemia, nosebleeds, cavities, cancer, loss of appetite, joint pain, wounds. It can be taken as a supplement or found in citrus fruits and natural juices.

Vitamin D: main function is helping Calcium and Phosphorous absorption. It is also involved in stabilizing the nervous system and maintaining proper coronary function. Found in milk, soy, fish, orange juice, and cod liver oil (my Grandfather used to give us this shit by the spoonful, but it was worth it).

Vitamin E: a fat-soluble vitamin essential for normal reproduction; an important antioxidant that neutralizes free radicals in the body. Antioxidants protect the cells of the body from the effects of free radicals, which have been known to cause cell damage which can contribute to the development of cardiovascular disease and cancer. Found in supplements, olive oil, egg yolks, and fish oils.

Feverfew: a traditional herb found in many gardens, Feverfew is commonly seen in the literature as, Chrysanthemum parthenium (L.) Bernh. and Pyrethrum parthenium (L.) Sm. Feverfew is used for reducing fever, for treating headaches (especially for migraine headaches) and for arthritis. Found around the world and in California.

Vitamin K: makes proteins for blood, bones, and kidneys. People taking blood thinning medicines, such as aspirin should limit their intake of vitamin K. There are three different forms of Vitamin K: phylloquinone, which is found in food, menadione, which is man-made and menaquinone, which is produced by the body. People who consume large quantities of alcohol are usually deficient in this vitamin. Vitamin K can be found in: green leafy vegetables, egg yolk, fruit, liver, and dairy.

Biotin: part of the B Vitamin Complex, Biotin helps the body use the Macronutrients from foods for energy. It aids the body in producing energy in the cells.

Pantothenic acid is needed to make cholesterol, bile, some fats, red blood cells, hormones and nerve regulators. Sources of biotin include dairy, meat, cereal, yeast, and also soybeans.

Folic Acid: this water-soluble vitamin and is one of 8 members of the B Complex Family and assists in the prevention of neural tube defects (spina bifida) in fetuses and also involved in production of brain chemicals like serotonin, that regulate appetite, mood and sleep. Found in fruits, vegetables and other foods.

Niacin: one of the eight B Complex Vitamins, Niacin works closely with vitamin B1, B2, B6, and biotin to break down the Macronutrients into energy. Good sources of niacin include grains, peas, beans, poultry, and meat.

Coenzyme Q10: this antioxidant has been found to have great effect on migraine headaches and is used to treat mitochondrial disorders and other metabolic disorders. Many people take Coenzyme Q10 to help improve heart function and to lower bad cholesterol levels. It is being investigated as a treatment for cancer and studies suggest that it protects the brain from Parkinson's and Stroke.

Fish Oil: especially Omega-3 oils are now considered a miracle for the human body. They can help prevent heart disease, lower bad cholesterol levels, control blood pressure, decrease joint pain, migraines, depression, autoimmune diseases, and improve perfect brain function.

Pantothenic Acid: this water-soluble vitamin is one of the few 8 B Vitamins that helps the body use Macronutrients from foods to produce energy in cells. Found in egg yolks, dairy products, legumes, etc.
Riboflavin: is also called Vitamin B2. Dairy products supply about 50% of the riboflavin that people receive. Aiding in physiological hypotrophy, Vegetarians are sometimes known to having riboflavin deficiencies due to lack of B Complex Vitamins. Found in dairy, meat, vegetables,   and   cereal.

Thiamine: known as Vitamin B1, it is needed maintain overall health. Thiamine is found in foods such as meats, brewer's yeast, dried beans, and peanuts.

Magnesium: Magnesium is a mineral that is abundantly found in nature, and the human body contains about one ounce of magnesium, mostly in bones and muscles. It can found in both plant and animal sources, though plants provide a richer source. It may be one of the most important anti-aging minerals, and magnesium is essential for calcium and vitamin C absorption, as well as helping the metabolism of phosphorus, sodium, and potassium. It helps convert blood sugar into energy and it is necessary for effective nerve and muscle functioning. It is often referred to as the anti-stress mineral. Many people are deficient in this mineral because of reliance on processed foods and because magnesium is easily depleted by none other than *stress*.

Iron: helps the blood and muscles deliver oxygen to every body cell, and it removes carbon dioxide from them. It is important to immune system functions, and the body self-monitors and regulates the absorption and use of iron for varying needs. Benefits include a provision of energy, stronger immune system, and proper mental function. Found in liver, red meat, baked beans, pork, soy, black-eyed peas, fish, chicken, oatmeal, rye bread, whole wheat bread, and juices.

Potassium: the third most abundant mineral in the body and is considered an electrolyte. It can help to prevent high blood pressure and may enhance the effect of antihypertensive medications. Both physical and mental stress can lead to a deficiency in potassium. Alcohol, coffee, and sugar can deplete potassium levels. It is vital to maintaining a normal heartbeat or heart rhythm. Potassium also functions and enables the body to convert glucose into energy, which is stored in reserve by the muscles and liver. Selenium: a mineral that fights diseases such as cancer and heart disease. It is a potent antioxidant that helps slow down aging. It is essential to many body functions and can be found in all cells, but more so in the liver, kidneys, spleen, and pancreas. Sodium: a mineral necessary for regulation of blood and body fluids, transmission of nerve

impulses, heart activity, and certain metabolic functions. Most people consume excess amounts, usually in the form of table salt and can have a dangerous effect on the health.

Zinc: plays an important role in cell division, growth, and repair. It helps with healing and maintaining a sense of taste and smell. It can be useful in fighting colds, flu, and other infections. Zinc is a component of over 200 enzymes, most of which are involved in protein and DNA synthesis. It has beneficial effects on sex and thyroid hormones. Found in crab, red meat, turkey, ham, pork, chicken, eggs, seafood, beans, split peas, cereal, wheat germ, and brown rice.

Amino Acids

In this section, we will address the main types of Amino Acids and their functions in the body. What are Amino Acids? They are organic compounds comprised of both an amino group and an acidic carboxyl group. They are the basic building blocks of proteins. There are 20 types of amino acids. 8 are considered "essential amino acids" that the body cannot produce and must be obtained from foods or supplements.

Alanine: one of the 20 amino acids commonly found in animal proteins, this amino acid contributes to fiber-strength, aids in stretching and flexibility. Alanine is not essential to the human diet, since it is synthesized from other cellular metabolites.

Arginine: one of the essential amino acids, it is abundant in histones and other proteins linked with nucleic acids. It is used as a dietary supplement for better water-solubility to proteins in neutral solution. It is also considered essential to the diet of children for optimum rates of growth.

Glutamine: a non-essential amino acid, its function is to regulate levels of toxic ammonia in the body can aid in the formation of Urea (excreted by the kidneys). It is also incorporated into proteins and is not essential to the human diet, since it can be synthesized from Glutamic   Acid.

Phenylalanine: an essential amino acid, Phenylalanine is found protein and is used in medicine/nutrition. It is one of the two amino acids making up Aspartame and contributes to the structure of the proteins in which it has   been   incorporated.

Tryptophan: another essential amino acid, it is found in small amounts in most proteins. It is important for growth and development and also used as a sleep aid (especially after eating turkey or drinking milk). It was recently   removed   from   the   market   in powder/supplement form, apparently due to a bad batch that possibly led to sickness in certain individuals.

Tyrosine: a non-essential amino acid, Tyrosine is a useful building block of protein. It can be manufactured in the body and is especially found in insulin. It is also a precursor of hormones.

Performance Supplements

Creatine: usually in powder form, helps maintain energy during a workout and faster recovery afterwards. Always follow directions on labels when using any supplement enhancer.

Protein Shake: they can play an important role for a person looking to gain muscle mass. There are many assortments of flavor, protein types (such as soy, egg, whey, and milk), brands, and quantities. Ask a health food store associate for information regarding proper selection. Some people may have difficulty digesting such shakes and should be monitored regularly. Weight Loss Supplements: in all honesty, some of these do help stop food cravings and burn off weight… mostly water weight. BUT they are sometimes more dangerous to a person's overall health and should be used with great care. As with any worthy goal in life, self-discipline and hard work will always result in greater rewards. A magic pill cannot replace will power in the gym. All diet and exercise programs start within each individual, not from external sources. If someone you are training with uses any of the afore mentioned, suggest that they always take with caution.

Healthy Foods

Sufficient water intake is needed by the body throughout the day, especially after a good workout. It makes sense, being that 70% of our body is comprised of water. Individual organs raise that estimate even higher, such as the brain which is approximately 80% water. If your client is concerned about adding water weight, let them know it's not from water! Instead, suggest that they omit soda, alcohol and other high calorie beverages from their diet.

Vegetables

<u>Asparagus</u>

<u>Avocado</u>

<u>Bell peppers</u>

<u>Broccoli</u>

<u>Brussels sprouts</u>

<u>Cabbage</u>

<u>Cauliflower</u>

<u>Celery</u>

<u>Collard greens</u>

Cucumber

Eggplant

Fennel bulb

Garlic

Green beans

Green peas

Kale

Leeks

Mushrooms, Crimini

Mushrooms, Shiitake

Mustard greens

Olives

Onions

Parsley

Romaine lettuce

Sea vegetables

Spinach

Squash, summer

Squash, winter

Swiss chard

Tomato, fresh

Turnip Greens

Root Vegetables

Beets

Carrots

Potatoes

<u>Sweet potato, with skin</u>

<u>Yam</u>

Seafood

<u>Cod</u>

<u>Halibut</u>

<u>Salmon</u>

<u>Scallops</u>

<u>Shrimp</u>

<u>Snapper</u>

<u>Tuna</u>

Fruits

<u>Apple</u>

<u>Apricot</u>

Banana

Blueberries

Cantaloupe

Cranberries

Fig

Grapefruit

Grapes

Kiwifruit

Lemon and Limes

Orange

Papaya

Pear, Bartlett

Pineapple

<u>Plum</u>

<u>Prune</u>

<u>Raisins</u>

<u>Raspberries</u>

<u>Strawberries</u>

<u>Watermelon</u>

Low Fat Dairy

<u>Cheese, low-fat</u>

<u>Eggs, hen</u>

<u>Milk, 2%, cow's</u>

<u>Milk, goat</u>

<u>Yogurt, low-fat, cow's milk</u>

Beans & Legumes

Black beans

Dried peas

Garbanzo beans

Kidney beans

Lentils

Lima beans

Miso

Navy beans

Pinto beans

Soybeans

Tempeh

Tofu

Nuts & Seeds

<u>Almonds</u>

<u>Cashews</u>

<u>Flaxseeds</u>

<u>Olive oil</u>

<u>Peanuts</u>

<u>Pumpkin seeds</u>

<u>Sesame seeds</u>

<u>Sunflower seeds</u>

<u>Walnuts</u>

Grains

<u>Barley</u>

<u>Buckwheat</u>

<u>Corn, yellow</u>

<u>Millet</u>

<u>Oats</u>

<u>Quinoa</u>

<u>Rice, brown</u>

<u>Rye</u>

<u>Spelt</u>

<u>Wheat</u>

Herbs & Spices

<u>Basil</u>

<u>Black pepper</u>

<u>Cayenne pepper</u>

<u>Chili Pepper, Red, dried</u>

<u>Cinnamon, ground</u>

<u>Cloves</u>

<u>Coriander seeds</u>

<u>Cumin seeds</u>

<u>Dill weed, dried</u>

<u>Ginger</u>

<u>Mustard seeds</u>

<u>Oregano</u>

<u>Peppermint leaves, fresh</u>

<u>Rosemary</u>

<u>Sage</u>

<u>Thyme, ground</u>

<u>Turmeric, ground</u>

Poultry & Meat

Beef, lean organic

Calf's liver

Chicken

Lamb, loin

Turkey, roast

Sweeteners

Blackstrap molasses

Cane juice

Honey

Maple syrup

Other

Green tea

Soy sauce (tamari)

Diet Theories

Low/No Carbohydrate Diets:

As stated earlier, in the past decade, there has been a surge in low carb popularity. The Ketogenic Diet (or Keto) consists of eliminating starches, sugars/carbs and even dairy (depending on the specific discipline). The science behind this diet is based on switching the body's energy source from sugar to fat (this process is called Ketosis). To achieve this state, it is recommended that a person consumes no more than 25 grams of net carbs per day. If you subtract dietary fiber from the total number of carbs on a food label, that provides the total net carbohydrates per serving. Eating leafy greens like spinach and kale or foods such as broccoli are considered safe in any quantity, because they do not raise the body's insulin levels. People on this diet avoid all foods containing carbohydrates, such as breads, pasta, potatoes, etc. Though it is helpful to keep carbs down, the amount should never fall below 50 grams per day when first starting out. It is safer to decrease carbs gradually; the human body is used to the energy that carbohydrates provide in order to perform daily activities.

The Carnivore Diet is more extreme in that only meat is consumed. Some keep cheese in their plan, while others omit all dairy due to its inflammatory nature. The same goes for processed foods like hot dogs, cold cuts and sausage- some continue to eat these foods, others cut them out completely. As of this writing, there hasn't been sufficient data to confirm or deny the safety of this particular diet. The brain also requires a sufficient amount of carbs in order to function properly. For a person who exercises, they should consume even more grams of carbohydrates each day. Another concern is that people on these diets are told they can eat whatever else they choose. To make up for the lack of carb-rich foods, they might overcompensate by eating a 16oz steak. Spiked levels of saturated fat and cholesterol can also be dangerous. Yet, when on such diets, it is important to eat enough vegetables or fatty cuts of meats to help digestion and avoid diarrhea.

Vegetarian/Vegan Diet:

Albert Einstein once said "Besides agreeing with the aims of vegetarianism for aesthetic and moral reasons, it is my view that a vegetarian manner of living by its purely physical effect on the human temperament would most beneficially influence the lot of mankind." Higher levels of animal protein can result in mood swings, but studies show that protein found in vegetables (such as soy) have a less severe effect. Too much soy can be binding and disrupt the digestive track at work. Consuming soy in moderation is best. Eating products such as soy nuts which are smaller in portion are easier for stomach acids to break down. The benefits of increased fruit/vegetable intake can aid in weight loss, vitamin optimization and better hydration. In contrast, vegetarians tend to lack the B complex vitamins which can only be found in animal foods. Supplements can be taken, but the B vitamins still come from animals. Some vegetarians (called Octo-ovo) may eat eggs and dairy, thus solving the B complex deficiency.

Low Fat Diet: for addressing cardiac health concerns, there is no better method than consuming low levels of saturated fats and cholesterol. The vegan diet is particularly useful here, but those who eat from animals should be aware of potential health concerns. Avoiding read meat is a plus. Ground beef prepared 90% lean can easily be found and excess fat can be sliced off. Eating chicken breast without the skin is better as well. Fish, such as salmon, has less saturated fat and cholesterol, but also contains the essential fatty acids (good fat) the body uses to function properly. Fats contain 9 calories per gram, which is the highest of the macronutrients.

Allergy Diet: many people suffer from various food allergies (i.e. lactose intolerance, peanuts, migraines, etc.). One some, the scent of peanuts from the other side of a room can result in an allergic reaction in the skin. Another person can eat chocolate and receive a horrific migraine. Others cannot eat dairy without the repercussions of stomach pain. Besides abstaining from these foods, there are methods such as the Rotational Diet, where vitamin C is increased along with the bioflavinoid quercetin. On the first day, the person is expected to fast and each following day, certain foods are added back into the diet. For most, this is the process of elimination. Most people are unaware as to what they are allergic to and this diet obviously helps them.

FDA Food Pyramid: the Food and Drug Administration provides a 5 level triangle chart that lists all food groups and suggested daily portions. Where this guide is limited in nature (servings vary with each individual food label, making it hard to calculate correct food pyramid portions), it is still the official government standard. At the bottom tier are the breads and grains (6-11 servings). The next level up consist of fruits/vegetables (3-5 servings for veg./2-4 fruit). Above this is meats and other proteins (2-3 servings). Fats and other "junk" foods cap off the pyramid at small quantities.

Glycemic Index

The Glycemic Index is a system for ranking carbohydrates based on their immediate effect on blood glucose levels. The glycemic index of a food is characterized by the area within the 2 hour blood glucose response curve (known as AUC) following the ingestion of 1 portion of carbohydrates. The AUC of the test food is divided by the AUC of the carb standard and multiplied by 100. Both the standard and test food must contain an equal amount of available carbohydrates. In other words, the GI is simply the measure of how the food your client eats affects their blood sugar levels.

It is important to note carbs that break down quickly have the highest glycemic index. These carbohydrates need less energy to be converted into glucose, resulting in rapid digestion and an increase of blood glucose. Complex carbohydrates that break down slowly have a lower glycemic index. This identifies slower rates of digestion and absorption of sugars and starches in foods. This method will be utilized in your business (especially in the area of weight loss), but make sure not to confuse your client. The goal is to have them understand the consequences of their diet to their blood sugar levels… without discouraging them.

Heart Rate

There are two ways of measuring heart rate. You can use a heart rate monitor, which will give you fast and precise results. These days, you can wear a monitor on your wrist (like a watch) and easily check it at any time. Always keep track of battery power, so your client doesn't freak out if there is no pulse reading. If you want to wait on using a monitor, you can also use your finger tips and press on your client's radial artery on the wrist. Make sure you never use their neck to check pulse count. During their exercise session, it is helpful to gage their heart rate by placing your index and middle fingers on their wrist and once you have found their pulse, count 10 full beats. Make sure you start counting their heart beats right after they stop the activity; you will only have a 15 second window of accuracy. Once you have obtained their 10 second pulse, multiply that number by 6. This determines their heart rate in beats per minute or what is known as BPM.

Age Target Heart Rate During Exercise

18-30	98-146	BPM
31-40	93-138	BPM
41-50	88-131	BPM
51-60	83-124	BPM
61+	78-116	BPM

Note: When selecting fruits and vegetables, it is always better to buy fresh instead of frozen and frozen is usually better than canned. Canned foods in particular, are highly processed and lose much of their nutritional value. On the plus side, they, like frozen foods, contain preservatives that keep them fresh longer.

Organic foods are becoming more widely available at major supermarkets and health food stores. For people worried about pesticides, they are all natural. Some claim that organic foods taste better than chemically enriched foods. Make sure these products have the "certified organic" seals on them.

The most important attribute a sports nutrition consultant can have, is the ability to observe. When consuming meat and poultry, always buy fresh and cook it thoroughly. Baking, broiling and grilling are the best methods of cooking; it is less fattening, but the nutritional value remains evident.

When buying cold cuts, remember that the meats have been restructured and contain added preservatives. This takes depletes their nutritional value in comparison to fresh meats.

The average percentage of body fat for men is 8-12% and 12-16% for women. The easiest way to measure is by: Under the skin is a layer of fat and the percentage of total body fat can be measured by using the thumb and the index finger and pick up the skinfold at selected points on the body and then apply a pair of calipers. Ensure that all of the skinfold measurements are located on the right side of the body and that the measurements are taken in millimeters (follow caliper instructions before applying to anyone!). You can also buy electronic devices that are accurate and easy to use.

Pregnant women should eat healthy and take vitamin supplements. Folic Acid (normally decreased with cooking) is important during pregnancy. Added vitamins will aid in healthier infancy and they also replenish the nutrients that absorb faster in the system.

Learn to read labels on all food and vitamin products! The Recommended Dietary Allowance (or RDA) provides the suggested amounts to consume daily. The United States RDA can be seen on many labels as well. This is the government's added measure of qualifying the RDA's procedures. Follow the recommended servings on all product labels, because each company manufactures their supplements differently.

Remind your client the importance of daily exercise. Though diet plays the most important role for overall health, exercise and nutrition work together for maximum   results.

Case Studies

Case study one:

"Amanda" came to me for nutritional advice. After I sat with and went over the Health Questionnaire she had filled out, I learned her goal was to lose twenty pounds, but she was concerned that she'd have to omit eating to do so. I explained to her that not only would "starving" herself be unnecessary, but in fact, it would also be counterproductive. The body needs proper nourishments to function correctly. When the body is lacking in the right nutrients, it will need to tap into muscles as an energy source. She smiled in relief as I continued to map out a daily diet that would correlate with her goals.

In order to maintain a body fat percentage between 12-16 percent, we needed to cut down on calories found in a lot of junk foods, soda, milk, cake, and breads. Obviously, foods high in fat like French fries and bacon were taken out, along with saturated fats in other foods she consumed. A great importance in breakfast was mentioned. I made her aware of the amount of protein she had been consuming- she couldn't lose twenty pounds, if she took in as much protein as a body builder. I suggested she cut out the late night snacks, because it'll pretty much sit in her stomach all night, while nothing is being done to burn it off. For breakfast, I recommended using egg beaters and make an omelet with mixed fruit. Since she couldn't stay away from cheese, I enlightened her on the miracle of Soy.

For lunch, a tossed salad with rice chopped up chicken breasts would go nicely with grape juice. For dinner, she could change it up with fish and celery sticks. If cholesterol is a factor, she might add carrots to her meals. Plain popcorn is a terrific snack. Since we're all different, I monitored her progression each week. If she lost too many calories, we added hot tea to her breakfast. She also cut sugar out of her routine. I told her that it was the worst food approved by the FDA. I saw a positive change in both her attitude and weight, which flattered me. I also received a large number of good quality referrals!

Case Study Two

After reviewing all of "Bert's" paperwork, I informed him that most problems young men have in gaining mass stem from their diet. I could see his frustration after working hard in the gym mainly revealed his lack of protein each day. He was surprised when I told him he really should eat one gram of protein for every pound he wants to weigh.

I introduced Creatine to his regimen and suggested he follow the loading directions on the label. I also suggested he try liver tablets, because they were used long before steroids and work well. The best time to take these additional supplements would be a half hour after a workout. For breakfast, I recommended he drink a big glass of O.J., cook about a dozen egg whites, toast a plain bagel, and take a multi-vitamin. Within three hours, take a soy protein shake, and possibly throw in a banana. For lunch, eat a 8oz lean steak, veggies, a couple of baked potatoes, and add three amino acids. Later, before dinner, add another shake.

Theoretically, dinner should be about the same as lunch. A substitution of chicken or fish, with a small portion of pasta is O.K. For desert, try half the amount of egg whites consumed for breakfast. It didn't take too long before he achieved his goal. I was happy to see how far he had come so fast. He put on about five pounds in two weeks thanks to this new diet alone! Now all he needs to do (besides continue his great progress) is smile now and then so the girls won't run away.

Case Study Three

I wanted to get a good feel of how well "Zack" would adjust to a low fat diet, knowing how new it was to his system. Without boring or confusing him, I explained the idea of a slow twitch muscle fiber type of program and healthier diet. Realizing his body fat is only pushing 10 percent, I wasn't as strict in my approach. I sensed skepticism, so I wanted to gain his trust first. We spoke between visits about different areas of interest. He, like me, enjoyed record collecting. That started us off on the right foot.

I mentioned the similarities to "Amanda's" nutritional scale and put him on a low fat diet. He was pretty lazy at first and I didn't want to upset him, so we agreed that he would follow this routine on the days we would meet: I taught him all about the Glycemic Index and how it measures the blood-insulin increases from certain foods (grape juice being one of the highest). For breakfast, I recommended using egg whites and make an omelet with mixed fruit. For lunch, a tossed salad was out of the question for him, so chicken breasts with corn and orange juice would do. For dinner, he didn't mind fish and rice. I always reminded him to drink plenty of water through out each day, to wash the excess garbage from his system. Since cholesterol was a factor, he cut out the beer during baseball on TV. No-fat pretzels and water were O.K. as a replacement. Being concerned of his mental state, I let him know that "No one is perfect. Don't kick yourself too much when you slip from your diet. Talk to me instead and together we can absolutely figure it out."

In the end, he continued working with me and made full time changes to his diet. Not only was he looking great, but his attitude improved a great deal. His posture improved dramatically and he began to feel   more   confident.

This completes the Sports Nutrition Certification section of the book. Once you are comfortable with the material, feel free to take the sample exam included.   Good luck!

CHAPTER THREE:

ADVANCED PERSONAL TRAINER

CERTIFICATION

What to expect

We will be covering all aspects of personal training, including:

Advanced Anatomy

Resistance Bands

Static (Isometric Training)

Isokinetics

Kickboxing Aerobics

Martial Arts

CrossFit

Pilates

Yoga

NOTE: *in order to successfully complete the Advanced Personal Trainer Exam, you will need to answer questions not only based on the new information listed above, but also on your previous personal trainer methodology (the advanced exam is cumulative).*

Advanced Anatomy

During your initial personal trainer certification program, you learned basic fundamentals concerning the human anatomy and how the major muscle groups interact with one another during exercise. You also learned about the three body types, muscle fibers and the affects of nutrition in our bodies.

At the advanced level, we will be covering a more in depth analysis of the human skelital system, coupled with joint movement, tendons, and how each functions during physical exersion. While studying this section (as with all portions of this text), be sure to take as much time as needed. It's not enough to temporarily memorize suitable definitions for the exam- in order to be a professional advanced trainer, you must come to *know* these funamentals.

Advanced Muscular Definitions:

Iliopsoas Muscle: a merger of two muscles, the Iliacus and Psoas, the Iliopsoas muscle ranges from the lumbar portion of the vertebrae to the femur. The main function of the Iliopsoas is hip flexion, lifting the thigh up towards the stomach region. This hip flexor also works in contrast- when stomach muscles move towards the thighs. Stomach crunches, leg raises and knee raises are common exercises that work this group.

Adductor Muscles: these muscles include the Adductor Magnus, Brevis and Longus, and the Pectineus and Gracilis. The Adductors begin at the pelvic bone and join at intervals along the extent of the femur. This connection provides power and firmness for the hip joint as well as the femur. Squats, lunges and adductions work these muscles the best. ****An adduction exercise is any that draws a limb inward toward the median axis of the body.*

Triceps Brachii: although you've already learned about Triceps, they actually have three heads called the Lateral, Medial and Long heads. The Lateral head is sited on the outward facing side of the Humerus (a <u>long</u> <u>bone</u> in the <u>arm</u> that runs from the <u>shoulder</u> to the <u>elbow</u>) and is responsible for the "horseshoe" shape of the Triceps. The Medial head is located along the center of the body. The Long head is toward the bottom side of the Humerus and is the largest of the three heads. Dips, pushdowns, and overhead dumbbell extensions are good for strengthening these muscles.

Rectus Abdominus: this abdominal muscle is known as the "six-pack" muscle of the abs. Many emaciated bands of tissue give it that appearance. Crunches, declined sit-ups and knee raises are good exercises for the Rectus Abdominus.

Transverse Abdominus: this muscle of the abdomen lies underneath all the other abdominal muscles and wraps sideways around the entire abdominal area. Lying leg raises, side bends and ball crunches strengthen this muscle.

Joints:

Every exercise involves the use of joints, whether your client is performing bench presses or curls. A joint is the location at which at least two <u>bones</u>

meet. They allow movement and provide structural support to bones, tendons, muscles, and ligaments. Bones are connected to each other structurally, but are also functional and anotomical.

There are three structural classifications of joints:

Fibrous Joint: connected by <u>fibrous connective tissue</u>.

Cartilaginous Joint: connected by <u>cartilage</u>.

Synovial Joint: not directly joined.

Joints are also classified functionally, based on mobility:

Synarthrosis: permits little or no mobility, such as in the skull.

Amphiarthrosis: permits slight mobility, such as in the spine.

Diarthrosis: permits great mobility, such as in the knees and elbows.

Joints are anatomically located in these groups:

Hands

Elbows

Wrists

Sternoclavicular Joints

Knees

Feet

Vertebrae

Hips

Temporomandibular Joints

Sacroiliac Joints

Ligaments & Tendons

Ligaments are connective tissues that clutch one bone to another, creating a joint. They control joint motion (i.e. stopping your elbow from bending backwards). Ligaments are comprised of strands of collagen fibers. Stretching increases flexibility of the muscles, although the ligaments do not actually stretch. They provide joint support so that we can perform maneuvers such as splits, high kicks and back bridges.

Tendons are made up of tough, fibrous tissue that connects a muscle with its bone. Similar to a sturdy bungee cord, Tendons can be flexible or tight depending on body movements. When a person stretches, the tendon becomes a tight cord. When an arm is bent, for example, the cord is loose and relaxed. They can also act as springs, working with muscles during exercises such as running. The Achilles Tendon absorbs shock during a stride, aiding the runner in energy conservation. Tendon length varies from person to person and is a considerable factor in gaining muscle mass. A person with shorter tendons and longer biceps will achieve better results compared to someone with longer tendons and shorter biceps. This is not to say a person in the second category cannot increase muscle size sufficiently- it may take more time than the first group and their overall gain may not be as large in proportion, but this is still just one factor in determining muscle atrophy.

Bone Anatomy

The human body consists of 206 bones (most of which are located in the hands and feet). You are not required to know all of these bones, nor will it benefit your clients. Having said that, as a fitness professional, it is important for you to have an elementary understanding of the major skeletal system. Not only will this knowledge offer specific insight when addressing a client's unique circumstance, but it also (from a business standpoint), looks impressive and more professional.

Bone Definitions

The Skull: the bony section of the head, the skull houses and protects the brain, while providing attachments for muscles of the head and neck. The *Cranium* is the top section of the skull, where the brain is located within. The *Mandible* is the jawbone connected to the skull.

Clavicle: also known as the *Collarbone*, the *Clavicle* is the long bone that makes up part of the shoulder and rotates along its axis when the shoulder is abducted. It is commonly injured in athletes and only takes about fifteen pounds of pressure to break.

Scapula: this bone forms the posterior part of the shoulder and is a flat bone, triangular in shape.

Sternum: or *Breastbone*. The *Sternum* is a long flat bone located in the center of the thorax or chest, connecting to the *Rib Cage*. Together they protect the heart, lungs and major blood vessels from injury.

Humerus: the long bone in the arm that runs from the shoulder to the elbow.

Vertebra: individual <u>irregular bones</u> in the spinal <u>column</u> (or *Ischis*). There are thirty three vertebrae in human beings, five of which fuse together forming the *Sacrum* (large, triangular bone at the base of the <u>spine</u>). *The Coccyx* or *Tailbone*, is the lowest section of the human <u>vertebral column</u>.

Pelvis: a bone structure located at the base of the <u>spine</u>, the *Pelvis* is formed by the <u>*Coccyx*</u>, the <u>*Sacrum*</u> and hip bones. There are differences between the pelvic region in men and women. The angle is greater than 90° in women and less than 90° in men. It is more heart-shaped in men and oval in women.

Radius: the main <u>forearm</u> bone that extends from the <u>elbow</u> to the <u>thumb</u> side of the <u>wrist</u>.

The Hand: made up of *Carpals* (actaully a part of the wrist), *Metacarpals* and *Phalanges*. *Carpals* are also known as *Wrist Bones* and consist of eight *Carpals* in each hand. *Metacarpals* are the five cylindrical bones extending from the wrist to the fingers. *Phalanges* are the actual finger bones.

Femur: or *Thighbone*. In <u>humans</u>, it's the biggest and strongest <u>bone</u> and can withstand up to 30 times the weight of an adult. It also forms part of the <u>hip</u> and knee.

Patella: or *Kneecap* is a large, triangular <u>bone</u> which works in conjuction with the <u>*Femur*</u> and protects the knee joint.

Tibia: the *Tibia* is the second largest bone in the body, located alongside of the *Fibula* around the calf.

Fibula: also known as the *Calf bone*, the *Fibula* is the outer and slimmer of the two leg bones.

Tarsus: the region between the leg bones and the *Metatarsus* (the five long bones of the foot connecting to the toes).

Resistance Bands

Resistance bands are an excellent addition to your personal trainer tool box- most people confuse these useful exercises with machine cables or they have no experience with them at all. Your client may need to adjust to the feel at first. Unlike free weights, where gravity used as the antagonist, resistance bands use consistent tension that makes movement feel awkward initially. They are cheap to buy and easy to set up. They also take up *very* little space.

Resistance band exercises are performed similar to regular methods, only they're positioned differently. Your client may stand directly on the band, gripping the handles for overhead presses and bicep curls. Bands can also attach it to doors for tricep pushdowns or wide angle lat pulldowns. They're great for balance work as well. Using them in conjunction with a Bosu develops coordination and strength.

You can easily load up your car with bands as opposed to lugging dumbbells to client homes and they give you and your client more variety. There are absolutely no limits to what you can do with them, as opposed to weights or machines. Finally, anyone can use them, whether they're just starting out or an experienced athlete in school.

Here are some really good exercises utilizing resistance bands:

Chest Press: with a band wrapped around a pole (a standing punching bag works too), have your client stand facing away from the pole while holding both handles. Have them keep the actual band cables under their armpits with palms facing each other. Next, have them squeeze their chest and press arms straight out in front of them in an even motion (about shoulder width apart at full extension). Slowly return to starting position, making sure to keep their chest tight throughout entire movement.

Rear Delt Row: ask your client to wrap a band around a pole, while sitting on a ball facing the pole. Holding the handles with arms straight out in front (palms down), have them pull their elbows back until level with their chest, while squeezing their shoulder blades.

Always keeping their arms parallel to floor, have them return to starting position.

Overhead Press: this one tends to be a bit awkward at first- make sure your client takes his/her time. Have them place both feet on the band and grip handles (this can be done either standing or seated on a ball for added balance work). They then lift hands up past their shoulders starting with elbows bent and palms facing in. Finally, have them return slowly back down.

Bicep Curl: here's a great bicep exercise- your client simply places both feet on the center of the band, while clutching handles and keeping both feet at least shoulder width apart. In a steady motion, have them tighten their biceps and bend their elbows, curling both hands up towards their front delts. Slowly return to starting position.

Squats: standing on the band with feet shoulder width apart, ask your client to grip both handles, in a bicep curl position at each side. Have them lower into a squat (using their buttocks to guide their motion), keeping their knees bent and back straight. They can pull on the band for added resistance. Slowly have them return to starting position.

Side Steps: this is excellent for the legs, glutes, thighs, and calf muscles. Have your client tie a resistance band around their ankles so that there are about six inches of band at standing position (feet should be hip distance apart). Have them take 10 steps to the left, tightening their thighs and glutes. Repeat on the right side.

Glute Kick: with your client on their hands and knees, ask them to wrap a band around their right foot. Holding the handles (with hands facing floor), have them extend their right leg straight back, squeezing the glutes in a even motion. Have them hold for a second, return slowly and repeat with their left leg.

NOTE: *if you are unfamiliar with resistance bands, make sure you practice these techniques before adding them to client work outs.*

Static (Isometric Training)

Static or *Isometric* training is an effective system of <u>exercise</u> where the practitioner contracts his/her muscle without any movement in the joint. This means the length of the muscle does not change, compared to *Isotonic* training where strength does not change but joint movement does.

Isometrics dates back thousands of years and was originally popularized in <u>*Yoga*</u> as well as <u>Chinese Martial Arts</u> (we'll be covering both systems later). Eventually, bodybuilders of the time implemented isometrics as part of their workouts. <u>Charles Atlas</u> favored this form of training and developed a group of exercises including isometric techniques. Unfortunately, the use of steroids began to tarnish the reputation of isometrics for muscle gain. When notable bodybuilders came under fire, the growth hormones used were then attributed to muscle increase- not isometrics.

Today, many people incorporate isometrics into their regimen, especially for strength training (not as much for muscle size). Good examples of specific isometric exercises include:

Isometric Rows: when using a rowing machine, your client simply holds the handles close to her chest squeezing the pectorals, in order to continuously put strain on the muscle. Repeat exercise 3 times.

Isometric Push Ups: have your client enter the classic push up position (arms extended, palms facing down). Have her lower herself about half way to the floor and hold position for 30 seconds. Remind her to contract all muscles for full effect. Repeat exercise 3 times.

Isometric Shoulder Raise: your client stands (feet shoulder width apart) and raises a light dumbbell directly out to the side. Once their arm is even with the floor, have them hold position for 30 seconds and slowly lower back to hips. Repeat exercise 3 times each arm.

Isometric Squats: with your client's back against the wall, have him lower himself until his thighs are even to the floor. Make sure his lower legs are even to the wall and his knees are bent. Holding his arms out in front, have him maintain this position for 30 seconds. Repeat exercise 3 times.

Isometric Calf Raise: while standing next to a chair, have your client stand on their right leg, keeping their left foot on the back of their right ankle. Have them stand on their toes and hold position for 30 seconds, using their hand on the chair for balance. Repeat exercise 3 times per side.

Side Bridge: beginning on her side, have your client push up with her right arm, pointing her left shoulder to the ceiling and legs fully extended (this should look like a longated body triangle). Have her hold position for 30 seconds, if possible. Repeat exercise 3 times per side.

NOTE: *when performing Isometric exercises, make sure your client breathes smoothly and consistently throughout the entire duration of position.*

Isokinetics

"What in the world is Isokinetics and how will it help me train people?"

The good news: you will come to fully understand what Isokinetics is… and what it is not. The bad news: once you have an accurate understanding of Isokinetics, you may never actually utilize it. You may be thinking, *"If I'll never use it, why do I have to know it?"*

The use of Isokinetic training has been available since the early nineteen seventies. It is an exercise performed with a particular machine so that no matter how much force is exerted, the movement takes place at a steady speed. It wasn't very popular at the time, based on its limited practices in rehabilitation. It was used primarily for exercise, but the machines were mechanically limited compared to today's standards. By the mid eighties, motor and microprocessor technology replaced early machines with superior equipment which, in turn, provided quicker results. Today, Isokinetics is a popular and trusted form of analysis in the medical field.

The problem with using Isokinetic machines, as opposed to a live partner, is the financial costs. A decent full body machine can set you back several thousand dollars, whereas a smaller foot pedal exerciser costs around $75 online (this device is most beneficial when working with senior citizens who have joint complexity). If you wish to incorporate Isokinetics into your client's regimen, it is strongly recommended that you work with natural human resistance unless purchasing a large machine is absolutely necessary. Again, if you work in a gym, there's a chance you'll have access to this equipment there. Otherwise, use your hands as resistance in a controlled motion, while your client pushes against you using either their own hands or clutch their ankles as they try to press upward from a seated position. Again, at this time, these tests are best used in determining your client's current strength and coordination only. If they are looking to gain muscle mass or wish to lose weight, Isokinetics is not the best method to achieve these goals.

NOTE: *while using minimal resistance, if your client goes completely limp and complains of numbness or pain, immediately stop the assessment and recommend he/she consults a physician.*

PLEASE READ BEFORE PROCEEDING: *Although the information in the following sections may not be your specialty areas, as an advanced trainer, you should have a basic understanding of these interests, as they are all <u>highly</u> popular means of exercise. Unfortunately, there are a great number of fitness professionals who lack this knowledge, despite the high demand from clients. For instance, if you are working with someone who expresses interest in adding Pilates to their regimen, you can help them decide if it's right for them, as well as help in choosing the appropriate program. Any detailed or historical information you provide will benefit them tremendously. Your professionalism will go a long way.*

Kickboxing Aerobics

Aerobic Kickboxing (also referred to as *cardio kickboxing*) has become one of the most popular methods of exercise in America. You can't find a gym in the US that doesn't offer some degree of kickboxing. It differs from other martial arts, in that fitness is the primary goal. It merges principles found in western boxing, martial arts and aerobics and is widely used by respected athletes for conditioning. Though this is not primarily used for self-defense, fluidity is paramount in BOTH martial arts and kickboxing aerobics. Also, unlike Muay Thai, kickboxing aerobics is non-competitive, so there is no sparring between partners. Kickboxing aerobics classes are usually made up of 10 minute warm-ups, 30 minutes of kickboxing and a 5 minute cool down period.

Kickboxing Techniques

Let's review some basics. A *repetition or rep* is a motion performed by lifting weight up from the starting position and down again. A series of repetitions performed is called a *set*. Two sets for the same muscle performed without stopping in between is called a *Super*

Set. When one larger set is performed without rest until all reps are completed, this is called *Circuit Training*. It is important to have a good understanding of these terms before training. Are you ready to kick some butt?

Basic Fighting Stance: standing with feet about shoulders width apart and knees slightly bent, the left arm comes up to protect the face (elbow bent). The right (or power) arm also comes up with hand next to right jaw line. With chin tucked in (it is the most vulnerable spot on the head), instill a rocking back and forth motion throughout the aerobics session. Keeping toes forward, turn torso towards imaginary opponent. Make sure to keep body loose and elbows pointing down (not outward).

Squat: bend each knee one at a time or simultaneously.

Toe Raises: stand up on the toes or balls of feet and come back down.

Marching In Place: in between any technique, it helps to keep blood circulating by marching in place. This can simply be an exaggerated and controlled walk, without moving in any direction.

Front Kick: raising either knee one at a time, kick same leg out in front in a snapping motion. Curl toes back so that the ball of the foot makes contact. Return back to high knee (or chamber) position and down again. Keep feet light during all kicks. Do not try to muscle power out of their legs. Knee Raise: lifting upward with the knee while contracting the abdominals.

Side Kick: similar to the front kick, only this time your hip turns outward and left foot pivots so your knee comes up on an angle. The key is to impact with the outside blade of the foot. Make sure your leg is horizontal with the floor. At first, you may kick lower. Always keep your hands up!

Roundhouse Kick: same as front kick, only pivot the front foot out and turn hips slightly while throwing the kick straight out. The shift in foot and hips will naturally cause the kick to whip on the right angle.

<u>Always</u> keep hands up until the actual kick. You can lower your right hand for better momentum.

Jab Punch: in fighting stance, the front arm punches straight out <u>while</u> the hips turn with it. The front foot also pivots out. This is where true power emanates from. A punch is useless without these movements. After impact, the arm retracts rapidly back into guard position. The punch should snap out.

Cross punch: in fighting stance, the rear (or power) arm punches straight out <u>while</u> the hips turn with it. The back foot also pivots out. This is where the true power comes from. After impact, the arm retracts rapidly back into guard position. The punch should snap out.

Hook Punch: in fighting stance, the front arm punches on a near horizontal angle with the floor <u>while</u> the hips turn with it. The front foot also pivots out. The key to this punch is that the hips should do the actual punch. The arm should remain stationary and let the body do the work. It helps to imagine carrying a broom over their shoulders and behind the head while swaying the waist back and forth. This punch may take some time to master, but it is well worth it!

Elbow Strikes: while rotating the waist, bend the elbows and swing out either horizontally or while squatting, launch in a vertical motion.

Knee Variations: in fighting stance, lift either knee into high chamber position straight up while contracting abdominal muscles. For a curved knee, pivot front foot out and turn hips with it. Then, return to fighting stance. Use arms as a "goal post" to swing through the knee strike. Always return arms to guard position.

Torso Twist: turn the torso forward or to either side or rotate the torso in a circular motion.

Straight or Bent Arm Extension: punch each arm straight out or bent in any direction while in motion.

Class Designs

If you are working out alone or with a client, follow these guidelines for maximum success. If you do not hold certification as a kickboxing aerobics instructor, use this information as reference only. To keep your training interesting, you can set up Shadowboxing stations (performing all techniques in the air to an imaginary opponent). This is great for balance and speed. If you train on heavy bags all of the time, you will never feel what is like to miss a target and get thrown off center. Incorporate the heavy bag to workouts for increased power and enhanced accuracy. For boxers, this also helps them to learn proper distance. Also, using a jump rope speed bag, punch mitts, and kick pads will keep anyone motivated! Make sure to safely train at all times.

Another difference between traditional martial arts and Kickboxing aerobics is the use of music in an aerobics class. Play music that is upbeat (100-150 beats per minute or BPM) during peak periods and slower music during warm up and cool down sections. Obviously, try not to select anything too fast, but make it something contemporary (though the occasional 70's disco can make someone's day).

Again, kickboxing aerobics classes are usually made up of 10 minute of warm-ups, 30 minutes of kickboxing and a 5 minute cool down period. You can eventually introduce light weight dumbbells and weighted ankle wraps to your program. Make sure to use no more than 2 lb. weights and spread out to avoid injury.

Kickboxing Pointers

Take it Easy at first! You do not need to launch full-blast kicks and punches in your first class. You should keep kicks low and try not to overextend.

Use boxing or MMA (mixed martial arts) gloves when hitting any object. Also, Mexican hand wraps are inexpensive and are widely used for hand protection.

In the beginning, start with 20 reps for each limb by counting up to 10 and then back down to 0. Use this method for each exercise. This number can be increased for advanced students.

You should dress comfortably, wearing sweat pants or shorts and a tee-shirt. Tank tops are fine as well. Sneakers are important in case of any debris on the floor.

At first, have no more than 3 kickboxing aerobics classes per week. It is perfectly normal to gradually build up one at a time. Remember, safety always comes first.

Enroll in an aerobics or kickboxing class!

If you become fatigued or dizzy, stop exercising and sit down. Drink plenty of water and find your breath. You should also stop for the day.

Make Use of jump rope drills, heavy bags, speed bags, punch mitts, kick pads, light dumbbells, and other training equipment. This will help condition and keep you interested. Also, don't be afraid to add pushups and bent knee raises to the warm up phase.

You are allowed to enjoy yourself and take pride in this great venture. Remember to have fun with it!

Pilates

Pilates is comprised of Western and Eastern techniques. The Western influence emphasizes strength, muscle tone, physical appearance, and motion. The Eastern approach seeks to develop harmony between body and spirit through concentration. When these main areas merge, the aim is to:

Strengthen the Center

Build Muscle Tone

Increase Body Flexibility

Lengthen the Spine

Total Body Efficiency

Origins

Joseph H. Pilates was born in Germany in 1880. He had suffered from various illnesses most of his childhood, such as Rickets, Asthma and Rhuematic Fever. In 1912, he moved to England and became a boxer. Shortly after, his involvement in World War Two led him into an Army hospital where he rehabilitated injured soldiers. It was during this period that Pilates, originally called *Contrology* had been formed. This aided in the recovery of wounded soldiers and many dancers eventually trained under Joseph. He had trained a boxer and the two moved to New York to fight and open the first Pilates gym. Joseph Pilates died in 1967.

Rather than performing many repetitions or reps of an exercise, Pilates used fewer, but more precise movements. He created more than 500 specific exercises. Each of these movements is executed without the use of weights (Pilates practitioners use their own bodyweight). He designed a system composed of 8 <u>Pilates Principles</u> that aid in strength, flexibility, awareness, muscle tone, energy, and improved concentration. Today, Pilates is used by Doctors and physical therapists in practice and has also become increasingly popular in the fitness industry. Research suggests Pilates can help in motor response, biomechanics, and musculoskeletal physiology.

Though just about anyone can use Pilates to improve themselves, it's benefits have been well established amongst athletes, dancers, senior citizens, pregnant women, obese people, and those suffering from chronic pain (especially lower back pain).

The Powerhouse

Created by Joe Pilates, it is the area between the bottom of the rib cage and the line across the hips consisting of the abdominal muscles, inner thighs, buttocks, back, and hip flexors. Since these are the main muscles of the lower torso, they are responsible for preventing back problems. When these stabilizers are well trained and developed, we place less strain on our backs and hips. The focus becomes the center, thus decreasing pressure on the spine and joints. Today, people sometimes refer to this principle as *core* training or stability.

8 Principles

Relaxation: in the beginning of every Pilates class, relaxing releases tension and resistence from our body.

Concentration: unclouded focus on each movement is to have control over your mind and body.

Alignment: the spine and surroundeing joints are straight and neutral, avoiding and correcting poor posture.

Breathing: the body needs oxygen to perform each exercise, so we must learn to breathe effectivily. Focus breath into the lower ribcage. Moving on the exhale enables core stability during each exercise and prevents *Valsalva* (breath holding). Long, fuller breaths help us to relax and remain calm during stress.

Centering: by targeting the navel with the pelvic floor (while properly aligned), we can achieve true centering. Little space between spine and navel essential.

Co-ordination: "Concentrate on the correct movements each time you exercise, lest you do them improperly and thus lose all the vital benefits of their value." – Joseph Pilates. The ability to stabilize one part while challenging another.

Flowing Movements: all techniques are fluid, graceful, in proper form, slow, and controlled.

Stamina: endurance, developed through consistent practice will keep you in tune in everyday life and in sports.

It is important to maintain precision and balance in all Pilates movements. Having a good understanding as to which muscles are to be isolated, which should become relaxed, where motion starts and stops, awareness of body positioning, and correcting bad habits (i.e. tightening of the jaw or shoulders). Through correct awareness, we develop *Muscle Memory* so our bodies will remember what it feels like to be in incorrect positions.

The Torso

Upper torso stability occurs anytime the arms are moving while the torso must remain still. The upper limbs challenge the torso to remain stable. Lower torso stability occurs anytime the legs keep the back from overextending or arching off the matt.

The Spine

The two main functions of the spine are to align the body (upright and strong) and allow flexibility. An enriched workout will engage both of these functions. Individual Pilates exercises will enable the spine to lengthen, by way of smaller muscles cushioning in between each vertebrae. When posture is poor, these muscle cushions wear down and lead to back injury.

<u>Pilates For Losing Weight</u>

Weight loss is generally accomplished through aerobic exercise and proper diet. For beginners, Pilates is a slower and low volume based method. Once a student becomes advanced, the workout levels increase and it turns into a high volume routine. It is recommended that a new student of Pilates who wishes to lose weight add a cardiovascular exercise to their weekly structure.

Pilates Techniques

I highly recommend taking Pilates classes from a professional first. If you are unable, I have listed some of the popular techniques used today. When practicing these or any other exercise techniques, make sure to move slowly and concentrate on breathing and maintaining proper form. It may take some time to become proficient, but if it were easy, the rewards would be smaller.

Neutral Spine: lying on your back, with knees bent. Your neck and lower back should not be touching the mat. This is to better absorb shock during activity.

Ballerina Arms: sit cross-legged and Straighten the spine as if leaning against a wall (notice the imagery). Bend the elbows at a 90 degree angle to protect the shoulder joint. Bring your arms back to connect the shoulder blades. Lower arms down so the shoulder blades slide down your spine. Raise the bent arms above your head (like a ballerina) and lower into starting position. Begin your sessions with 1 set of 3 reps.

The Roll Up: lie on your back with legs straight and arms stretched above your head, shoulders down. Keep your back flat on the mat and slowly lift your arms toward the ceiling as you inhale. As you exhale, slowly roll forward, lifting your spine off the mat. Keep your head straight forward and stomach stretched. Inhale once again, stretching out over your legs. Exhale while slowly rolling back down to the mat. Do up to 5 reps.

Bridge: lie on your back with knees bent, feet flat on mat. Push hips upwards and hold. Keep your navel in towards your spine, but your torso should be well aligned (not bent). Slowly lower your hips down to the mat. Repeat this 3-4 reps.

Bridge on Exercise Ball: lie on your back with legs straight, calves flat on ball. Push hips upwards and hold. Keep your navel in towards your spine, but your torso should be well aligned (not bent). Slowly lower your legs down on the ball. Repeat this 3-4 reps.

The Hundred: lie on your back, arms at your sides. Bend knees into chest, while drawing chin towards knees. Do not lift your head past shoulders. Slowly return to starting position.

The Saw: sitting up straight, with legs out in front, reach arms out to both sides. Reach your left arm down over your right leg. Your spine should roll as you descend.

Once your hand is near the floor, chop your foot lightly 3 times and flex your buttocks. Switch to other side.

C-Curve: sit up straight, legs slightly bent. Envision a ball hitting you in the stomach. Your spine becomes curved, while shoulders remain straight. This works your abdominal muscles. Once your body is curved like the letter C, slowly return to starting position. Repeat up to 5 reps.

The Swan: lie on your stomach with head on the mat, arms up in front on a roller (palms facing each other in a blade position). On the exhale, pull the roller towards you, raising your head and neck off the mat. Aim your chest for the sky, following your head. Keep hips down on the mat. Slowly lower roller to starting position. Repeat 3-4 reps.

Arm Reach/Circles: lie on your back, knees bent. Inhale, while stretching your arms to the sky. Hold for a second, then exhale while bringing your arms back behind your head. Keeping your lower back down, widen your arms back down (like slow snow angels) and end up in starting position with arms out in front. Repeat up to 10 reps.

Cat Stretch: while on all fours, knees should be under hips and hands under shoulders with palms flat. Contract the abdominals to bring the head, neck and back in alignment. Inhale and bring the hips towards the ceiling while drawing the shoulders back and away from your head. Look straight up. Exhale while tucking the chin and pulling your navel towards your spine. Round the back and slowly return to starting position. Repeat 4-6 reps.

Inner Thigh Stretch: sit on the floor and extend your legs in front of your body. Bend your knees, feet together flat on the floor. Place your hands on your calves Slowly let your knees fall open to each side and slide the soles of your feet together. Rest your hands on your ankles. Slowly round your spine and roll your shoulders forward. Lean forward, lowering your upper body toward your legs. Stop when you feel the stretch in your _inner thighs_. Return to starting position. Repeat up to 10 reps.

When practicing Pilates, it helps to use visuals to correct posture issues. Similar to metaphor, these images can paint a realistic landscape anyone can utilize. For instance, when lengthening the spine, one might emphasize tuning a piano chord and so on. Be creative!

Yoga

Yoga is said to have originated in India over 26,000 years ago. The goal of yoga was to ascend out of disease and suffering and into enlightenment. This was known as "Samadhi." The practice of yoga leads to a profound understanding into the nature of all consciousness. Around 600 B.C., the practices of yoga (or the Eight Limbs of Patañjali's Yoga) were written by Patanjali in India and spread across the globe. Yoga can also be linked with Tibetan Buddhism, where practitioners ultimately evolve into the highest level, "Ati yoga."

Eventually, students of yoga are to achieve enough understanding of the techniques so that they may acquire the fundamental yoga of freedom, a state that is known today as "Super-mind." In my experience with yoga, I have benefited tremendously from breathing conditioning, the many inimitable stretches involved and exceptional muscle strengthening postures.

Benefits of Yoga

Weight Loss

Tone

Increased Health

Flexibility

Better Posture

Calmness

Inner Peace

Mental Concentration

Strength

Balance

Coordination

Rejuvenation

Energy Expansion

Yoga Types

There are various forms of yoga, but three of the most popular types are: Hatha Yoga, Power Yoga and Bikram Yoga. Hatha is the most trained form of yoga today. Power Yoga is a more aerobic in nature, with a strong base in cardio. Bikram is a style of yoga practiced in a heated room in order to hasten detoxification. These are the three types of yoga that you will most likely discover. Other styles of yoga intended for fitness minded people are Iyengar Yoga and Ashtanga Yoga. These provide higher levels of intensity for the advanced practitioner. Sivanda Yoga and Kripalu Yoga both incorporate meditation, psychology and health sciences.

Yoga Poses and Techniques

Yoga poses or *Asanas* are comprised of several combinations of stretching and breathing. They're classified into numerous types depending on the posture and the consequential benefits. Some concentrate on specific parts of the body, while others encompass the entire organization. These poses can be classified into positions, bends, balance techniques, twists, supine and prone poses, and inversion and relaxation poses.

Positions

Mountain pose (Parvatasan) is considered to be the most fundamental standing pose and central to forming other asanas. It's intended to assist legs and hips for improved posture. Benefits of standing positions are strong leg muscles, increased mobility in neck and shoulder and superior flexibility in the lower back. *Lotus Pose*

(Padmasana) is a basic seated pose and is used in numerous asanas. There are primarily two seated poses, one with legs crossed and other with legs folded back. These poses are good for strengthening the back and hips. They present dexterity to spine and flexibility to hips, groin, knees, and ankles. Combinations of deep breathing, normal breathing, fast breathing, and breath control in the seated position are used for attaining inner calmness and decreasing breathing related problems.

Bends

Back bends strengthen the shoulders, chest, rib cage, and arms. This results in the comforting of the frontal body and improving the firmness of the spine. Correctly executing back bends can help reduce backache and shoulder pain. Forward bends are beneficial for strengthening the lower back, spine, shoulders, and neck. Bend positions are designed for attaining a sensation of relaxation and calmness.

Balance

Balance or *Santulan* poses are implemented for

improving muscle tone, body posture, concentration, and coordination. It aims at strengthening the spine, enhancing balance and building stamina.

Twists

These poses, when performed properly, help to release tension and stiffness throughout the body. They are practiced on both sides of the body and result in improved shoulder and hip mobility and spine elasticity.

Supine

Supine poses are performed lying on your back and ideal for improved abdominal and hip muscles and better spinal mobility. In several combinations, the body is either kept flat on the floor or can be lifted up from the floor entirely (or partially with the support of hands or legs or both). Prone poses are performed facing the floor. These poses help strengthen shoulders, arms, spine, and legs. They also aid in relaxing the lower back and are used to remedy backaches. In some cases, upper and lower parts of the torso are extended and lifted upwards, fully supported by the abdomen.

Inversion

These poses are performed keeping the legs at higher location than the chest. This leads to better blood circulation in the upper body. Possibly the most famous asana from this pose is *Sheershasana*, where the body is suspended upside down for several seconds.

Relaxation

These poses are used to calm the body and mind after practicing other poses. They help to cool the body down and reach mental neutrality.

Since the beginning, there have been numerous modifications and additions to yoga. All poses can be used successfully for healing ailments in conjunction with medicine, as well as fitness acceleration and stress reduction. Check your local papers and library for upcoming classes.

Martial Arts/Qigong

I've included this section as a bonus, not only because of my personal experience in MA, but also due to its increasing popularity in fitness. Throughout history, millions of people have reaped the benefits martial arts practice. Currently in the United States, mixed martial arts (or MMA) have surged in popularity. There are many excellent reasons to sign up at your local dojo. Whether your clients are looking to get in the best shape of their lives, cope with stress better, overcome anxiety, increase self-confidence, learn to defend themselves, or make friends, now is *definitely* the time! Again, this information should only be used for reference. If you are not ranked as an instructor, the knowledge you gain from this section will still be of great assistance for any client starting out, but isn't sure what style to choose (or what to expect in class).

Origins of the martial arts vary depending on various styles.

Most historians credit Qigong/Shaolin Kung Fu's origins to an Indian monk named Tat Moh, (known as Boddhidharma). As a Buddhist monk, he traveled much the world and taught Buddhism in different monasteries. In the year 520 A.D. Tat Moh finally settled at a Chinese monastery called Shao Lin (little forest). He found the monks to be weak and decided to live in seclusion for nine years. It was during this time, he had developed sets of exercises that would later be taught to the monks.

As the monks became more proficient in these Yoga types of techniques (which are systems commonly referred to as Tai Chi and Qigong), their vitality also improved to outstanding levels. To further protect themselves from bandits, the monks traveled to monasteries and taught fighting movements based on Tat Moh's principles. Since Buddhist monks are gentle and peaceful, their new fighting system was created *only* to defend themselves against an attack. The Lohon style is the earliest known form of Kung Fu, based on Temple Lohon. It is considered to be a simple form, comprised wide, well-rooted stances and powerful strikes.

This spawned an evolution in forms, including the Tiger Style (created by a Chinese emperor), the Tai Chor style, the 5 animal style, Hung Mei Pai, Tai Chi, and countless other variations. It's important to note that all Kung Fu and Tai Chi emanated from Qigong: "Qi" or "Chi" from Tai Chi and "Gong" or "Kung" from Kung Fu. Today, Qigong is known primarily for its health benefits. By cultivating your Chi (life force) through specific slow movements and breathing patterns, overall circulation and blood flow improves.

In the late 1960's, a popular movie star named Bruce Lee helped increase Kung Fu's demographic. Before his untimely death in 1973, he had developed a philosophy known as Jeet Kune Do. This has been considered to be the first mixed martial art, despite great controversy concerning it's understanding. Though some of the original form of Kung Fu has been lost, there are many traditional schools practicing throughout the world today.

There are no shortages of theories concerning the history of Jujitsu. The most accepted of these theories takes us to the feudal days of Japan. Some believe Jujitsu can be traced back 2,500 years when the name Jujitsu (or Gentle Art) hadn't been used. Many titles have been associated with Jujitsu, including taijitsu, kempo, toride, judo, yawara, kogusoku, wajitsu, aiki, shukaku, hakuda, kumiuchi, and more. It is said that there are over 700 different forms of Jujitsu and most have died with the families who practiced them. In fact, Jujitsu was considered to be a private art only taught within families. You may ask "Why is it called a gentle art, if people get hurt?!" The best answer to that question lies in the heart of the Samurai. Considering these warriors had to fight to the death with swords, Jujitsu could certainly be considered soft in comparison. Also, ancient practitioners mainly utilized joint locks and throws that were designed for total control of an assailant. This contrasts other means of self-defense, such as Karate and western boxing, in that punches and kicks are used more so to stun or set up finishing holds. On the contrary, Jujitsu has expanded through the years and variations have implanted the use of strikes regularly.

No one knows for sure who founded Jujitsu, but the story that is widely known deems Chin Gempin as the creator. He was a Chinese who became a Japanese subject from 1659 until his death in 1671. While at the Kokushoji temple in Tokyo, he taught jujitsu to three ronin (samurai discharged from duty). Shichiroyemon Fukuno, Yojiyemon Miura and Jirozayemon Isogai had learned from Gempin and eventually founded their own schools of jujitsu. Some disagree that he had started Jujitsu, saying it was born in China. Others believe the Takenouchi-ryu system founded in 1532 is the source of Japan's jujitsu forms.

Over time, Jujitsu has spread throughout Asia, later into North and South America. In 1914, Master Mitsuo Maeda migrated from Japan to Brazil and taught political leader Gastao Gracie's son Carlos techniques from Judo and Japanese Jujitsu. Over time, Carlos shared his techniques with his family and Gracie Jiu-Jitsu was born. It has become a highly respected system of self-defense, where a smaller, weaker person can overcome an attacker twice their size. The most effective techniques are various submission holds, such as the arm bar, triangle choke, kimora, and Americana.

A person can win a fight from his/her back utilizing the guard position or from the top mount, rear, standing, or side positions. BJJ is used for self-defense and sport tournaments.

Speaking of sports combat, Judo has become one of most proven forms of martial arts. Jigoro Kano lived in Mikage, a small town in Japan and was very sick as a boy. He decided to do something about it, when he enrolled in the Tenjin Shinyo ryu school of Jujitsu. Eventually, he studied at the Kito ryu school where techniques were supple and dealt more in free-form throws. Although he always showed respect for his masters, Kano sought after more philosophical reasons beneath his martial arts training.

In the late nineteenth century, Kano omitted all striking from the techniques he had learned and created his own system consisting of throws and joint locks. At only twenty two years old, he developed a sport called Kodokan Judo (a place to study the way). Kano finally established the first Judo school, called the Kodokan, in Tokyo. Today, millions of people visit this school each year! In 1886, there became great rivalry between Jujitsu and Judo schools, so a contest was held to prove which was superior. Kano's students won.

In the 1964 Olympics, Judo was first introduced as an official sport and became famous worldwide. By 1982, the Kodokan had established sixty five Judo techniques and ultimately incorporated weight categories to the sport. Today, children are taught the art of Judo- something that was once considered too dangerous. In certain clubs, Kata is also practiced as means of self-discipline and control. Though it is considered an excellent form of self-defense, Judo is probably best known as a competitive sport.

Although Karate can be linked back to Boddhidharma's teachings, it's distinction from Kung Fu first surfaced in Okinawa. The main island in a set of Ryuku Islands, Okinawa was considered a large trading route. Aside from nobles bringing metals, foods and wine, the teachings of martial arts also passed through.

Karate or *empty hand* was a native form of fighting, in part due to bans on weapons. In each city, anyone from kings to fishermen learned self-defense techniques, which were known as *Okinawa-Te* until eventually separated into three groups: Shorin-ryu (which is still popular today), Tomari and Shorei-ryu. Today, there are four main systems of Karate. Shotokan, founded by Gichin Funakoshi in early 20th century, Goju-ryu, founded by Chojun Miyagi (this name may ring a bell for movie goers), Shito-ryu, founded by Kenwa Mabuni, and Wado-ryu, developed by Hienori Otsuka from Jujitsu and Karate. The movements of Karate are based on well rooted stances, hard blocks and both open handed and closed fists strikes. Kicks are generally sharp and direct in function, not quite as "flashy" as in Tae Kwon Do. Kata was instilled as a simulated response to multiple attacks. Its purpose is to enhance form and self-discipline. The vocal release of the "Kiai" sound is used to generate power when striking and also to intimidate opponents.

Tae Kwon Do began in Korea during the Koguryo Dynasty (37 BC - 668 AD). Murals painted on the walls of warriors' tombs illustrate men fighting, though it was different than modern day Tae Kwon Do. The evolution continues with each new generation.

The Sonbae was a corps formed to protect Koguryo from enemies. Their training practices eventually spread to the Silla Kingdom where new methods were incorporated. In 537 AD, King Jin Heung revered what was then known as Hwarang (or Flower Knight) a fighting system that aided in unifying the Korean peninsula during his time. several years later, King Yoorie held Soobakhee contests. Although they were a ritual of prayer, the hand and foot techniques showcased have been considered to be precursors to today's movements.

By mid 20th century, many different names were associated to these practices until they finally merged in 1955. Tae Soo Do (sometimes used today), was the title for about two years, when the name Tae Kwon Do had been adopted. General Choi Hong-hi had implemented Tae Kwon Do as an integral part of police and military training. Under his rule, the Korean Tae Kwon Do Association (KTA) was established in 1965. Shortly after reaching America, the KTA became the World Tae Kwon Do Federation, which became an Olympic sport in 2000. Tae Kwon Do is most notably distinguished from other styles due to advanced kicks and competitiveness throughout the world.

Traditional kickboxing has been around for centuries. Muay Thai can be dated as far back as 2,000 years, originating in what is now China. It was once considered the sport of kings, used when King Sen Muajng Ma died and his sons fought each for the throne. Eventually, every soldier learned Muay Thai and continue practicing today. Certain kings from the Ayutthaya period were known as Muay Thai champions. Phra Buddha Chao Sua known as the "Tiger King" dressed as a peasant in order to fight (it was improper to touch a king). He won a prize of one baht and eventually defeated the national champion.

Competitive kickboxing in the United States started in the mid to late1960s, when black belts in various styles engaged in full contact competitions. Protective head gear and gloves were worn for safety and a point system was generally instilled. Today, kickboxing (along with mixed martial arts) has become popular on TV and live shows around the world.

Etiquette

Regardless of which martial arts system that most appeals to your client, there are universal laws that must be practiced and obeyed. Here's a list of common practices that should help you decide whether martial arts training is right for your client. While every school is different, these fundamentals should be valued wherever you go.

THE WARDROBE MAKES THE WARRIER

Ok, maybe I'm pushing it here. The truth is, most traditional Dojo's require all students to where a uniform or "Gi" to each class. They vary in texture and contain colored belts to show rank (usually from white to black). Some believe that rank was determined by how dirty the belt became. In other words, the more experienced the student, the darker his belt turned. Others disagree with this claim. Today, some schools are more informal in this area, allowing students to train in tank-tops and fight shorts.

THOU SHALL TRAIN, NOT STRAIN

The most important focus when exercising is "safety first." During all phases of learning (whether your belt color is white or brown), each student is expected to pay close attention to instruction at <u>all</u> times. Under no circumstance will any boasting or fooling around be permitted in class. Showing off techniques is a distraction to the class and also dangerous. Whereas challenging ourselves is paramount to success, overexerting can lead to personal injury.

Always practice using caution and be patient when working with partners.

THOU SHALL RESPECT THY PEERS... AND THY INSTRUCTORS

Regardless of discipline, we are all to treat and be treated as family. There will be no black sheep amongst us (just black belts). We are all unique individuals and deserve to be respected equally. If someone in class insults or physically harms you or a fellow student, please speak to your Sensei (teacher) right away. We are here to help each other grow, not compete against our egos.

TO BOW ONE'S HEAD IS TO BE HUMBLE.

Upon entering and exiting the room, many schools expect you to bow towards your class (and sometimes to a shrine). This shows respect to your teacher, students and school. During all class demonstrations, each student is required to remain silent unless a question arises. Remember: martial arts training is about kindness, respect and maturity.

TARDINESS IS NOT IN FASHION

Showing up to class on time is not only imperative to achieving martial arts goals. Learning to become more punctual aids in self-discipline and demonstrates our dedication to all areas of life. There will be times when uncontrollable events take place, forcing us to be late. That's OK. Simply bow-in and quietly join the group. If you cannot make a class, that's OK too. If you miss a few, don't get discouraged. Life happens to all of us… just come back stronger!

HATH THOU HEARD THE SAYING "MARTIAL ARTS TRAINING IS FOR SELF DEFENSE ONLY?"

Well, it's true. Although each is a system comprised of various fighting techniques and even hold tournaments, always remember your founder's intentions. Challenging ourselves is productive, competing with others can be beneficial or destructive. The honors we receive through training are found <u>within</u> each of us, not from external sources of exhibition. Again, Martial Arts training is not about hurting people- it's about working towards our full potential as human beings.

IF IT IS NOT ENJOYABLE, IT'S NOT AN ART

This can only mean one thing: HAVE FUN!

Martial Arts Techniques

It is difficult to learn martial arts from a book. Even instructional DVDs cannot replace the teacher/student relationship, although they can be effective. Each style has a unique set of principles (i.e. some schools will teach you to chamber your blocks, while others utilize a classic boxing guard), so it would be unfair to list instructions for any. Instead, I have compiled a broad list of sample techniques taken from various systems. *I do not condone the practicing of throws or submission holds without proper assistance.*

Break Falls/Rolls

Fighting Stances

Blocks

Footwork

Strikes (i.e. punches, kicks, elbow, knees, etc.)

Grappling/Submission Techniques

Self Defense Techniques

Sparring/Grappling

Multiple Attackers Defense

Weapons

CrossFit

CrossFit has become a popular form of exercise around the world. It is estimated that over 7,000 gyms in the United States have implemented this program to offer additional training options for customers. It consists of a high intensity variety of aerobics, weightlifting and calisthenics. Daily performance is typically rated by WOD (Workout of the Day) and most equipment utilized can be found in your average gym including kettlebells, plyo boxes, climbing ropes, mats, etc. Athletes incorporate CrossFit into their regimen to better develop coordination, balance, speed, strength, stamina, flexibility, power, accuracy, agility, and endurance.

Unfortunately, there has been great controversy concerning CrossFit in recent years. As for injury rates, statistics vary from 20% of practitioners up to 4 times that amount. In a recent survey by Hak and colleagues, out of 132 participants, 73.5% sustained injury from engaging in CrossFit. Needless to say, the safety of your client should be your first concern. Potential liability should be your second. As of this writing, there is a myriad of negative information concerning this method of training. Until more positive data becomes available, I recommend merging high intensity cardio with weight training methods listed prior. With creativity, you can help your client achieve similar results during sessions.

This completes the Advanced Personal Trainer Certification section of the book. Once you are comfortable with the material, you may take the sample exam. Good luck!

SAMPLE FORMS

<u>Health Questionnaire</u>

1) Do you have any history of heart problems?

2) Have you had any major surgery (back, knees, hip, etc.)?

3) Do you have a history of high blood pressure and/or cholesterol?

4) Do you experience chronic pain in your back, neck, shoulders, or other areas?   If so, in which areas?

5) Do you have any joint, muscle, or bone ailment (arthritis, osteoporosis, carpal tunnel, etc) which could be worsened by exercise?

6) Are there any other reasons, physical or psychological, that may inhibit your ability to safely participate in an exercise regimen?

7) Are you over the age of 65?

8) Are you under the age of 21?

9) Why are you seeking a professional trainer?

10) How much do you exercise each week?

If you said "yes" to any of the above health concerns, you should consult with your doctor. He/She can then determine if you are well enough to follow through with our exercise program. We will gradually be increasing your level of activity; therefore, your doctor must be aware of and comfortable with any such changes to your regimen. If your doctor knows of the health concerns listed above, please initial your answer. Also, give a short explanation as to why you and your doctor have decided you are fit to proceed with the regimen.

Name:___________________________________

Date:______________

Signature:______________________________

Release Form

I, ___________________________, understand and agree to the terms and conditions of this release form on this date________________ in the year ______________. As a voluntary participant in these activities, I am fully aware of the risk of injury that accompanies any kind of physical exercise, change in diet, use of exercise equipment, and physical training and instruction; therefore, I take full responsibility for proceeding despite this known risk. I agree to release (blank) from any claims, lawsuits, liabilities, and responsibilities for any such injury resulting from these activities. I also agree to consult with my regular physician before undertaking or changing this or any other exercise program.

Name:____

Date:________________

Signature:_____________________________________

Sample Exams

FINAL EXAM FOR

Personal Trainer Certification Course

This test contains multiple choice and true/false questions (75 total points) as well as an essay (25 total points). Make sure you have studied the book thoroughly before taking this exam. Simply skimming the text for answers will only hinder your confidence as a trainer and may present dangers to your client.

A grade of 85% is required for passing. Work hard and **GOOD LUCK!**

FULL NAME:
MAILING ADDRESS:
PHONE NUMBER:
EMAIL ADDRESS:

(Choose the Most Appropriate Answer)

1. Weight loss = high volume, low intensity exercise. Muscle building = high intensity, low volume exercise.

TRUE
FALSE

2. When setting up a legal business structure, you will need:

A. Corporate press pass

B. $30,000 in capital

C. A tax identification number

D. Someone to co-sign a lease

3. The muscles of the neck are called the:

A. Neck flexors

B. Sterno Mastoids

C. Gastrocnemous

D. Quadriceps

4. Anaerobic:

A. Incorporates weight training

B. Focuses on distance runners

C. Is a micronutrient

D. All of the above

5. Protein contains 9 calories per gram and has the most calories of all macronutrients.

TRUE

FALSE

6. High volume training is:

A. High intensity

B. Low intensity

C. Performed with loud music

D. Requires "train to failure" approach

7. The Ectomorph body type is:

A. Naturally muscular

B. Usually thin

C. Obese in certain areas

D. Both A & C

8. Slow twitch muscles are best trained using __________ weight.

A. Heavier

B. Resistance

C. Lighter

D. Dumbbells

9. To add muscle mass, clients should consume more:

A. Fat

B. Beer

C. Protein

D. Vitamins

10. A strong marketing plan should include:

A. Webdesign

B. Business cards

C. Ads in papers

D. All of the above.

11. When training your abdominal muscles, it is important to isolate the different sections (i.e. upper and lower abs) by using different exercises.

TRUE

FALSE

12. Lifting heavier weight between 12-25 repetitions results in larger gains and is the most beneficial formula for building muscle mass.

TRUE

FALSE

13. A good motto for a personal trainer to endorse is:

A. Train, don't strain

B. Weights get dates

C. No pain, no gain

D. None of the above

14. The Deltoids are responsible for raising the arms to the sides and overhead.

TRUE

FALSE

15. Anaerobic movement requires oxygen, which occurs during high volume, high intensity exercise.
TRUE
FALSE

16. When establishing heart rate, you should only use the wrist and neck.

TRUE

FALSE

17. The most common scenario you will encounter is a person trying to lose weight and tone up. Let's assume "Margarita" is a healthy 38 year old woman. Which of the following can she use to attain her goals?

A. Step aerobics
B. Weight training

C. Low fat diet

D. All of the above

18. Elements of exercise include all of the following except:

A. Isotonic

B. Coordination

C. Explosiveness

D. Micronutrients

19. When performing the one arm dumbbell row, make sure your client's back is curved enough to keep from straining too much.

TRUE

FALSE

20. _______________ is actually made up of muscles in the upper back *also* involved in pulling weight inward and holds the arm and shoulder together.

A. Extensor Capri

B. Pectoralis Minor

C. Rotator Cuff

D. Gastrocnemeus

21. For all exercises, tell your client to inhale slowly during contraction and exhale during release.

TRUE

FALSE

22. The most important attributes a personal trainer can have, is the ability to speak, command, and observe.

TRUE

FALSE

23. "Chester" is a 22 year old male who is desperately trying to add 20 lbs of muscle mass. He has worked out in the past, but his body responds like a rubber band. Which of the following would *not* help him increase muscle hypertrophy?

A. Protein shake

B. Running

C. Lifting heavier weight

D. Salmon

24. You are starting your own personal training business. In the beginning, it is recommended that a trainer offers rates of $45-65 per hour or $25-35 per half hour sessions.

TRUE

FALSE

25. Since you are not a medical professional, CPR certification isn't necessary for you to possess.

TRUE

FALSE

26. Carbohydrates are made up of compounds containing_________ and the types include_________.

A. Carbon/sugars
B. Hydrogen/water
C. Starches/air

27. The most popular occurrence for a self-employed trainer is traveling to your clients homes.

TRUE

FALSE

28. High intensity exercises include:

A. Bench press
B. Stair climber
C. Dead lifts,

D. All of the above

29. Motivation is paramount to the success of every personal trainer. Based on this statement, ______________ is the *most* important ingredient in developing lasting motivation.

A. Belief
B. The unconscious mind
C. Diet and exercise
D. Acceptance

30. If you can dream up negative and destructive circumstances, you can also dream up positive and constructive alternatives.

A. TRUE
B. FALSE

31. ______________ body structure is characterized by having broad shoulders, naturally larger muscles, thin waists, and faster metabolism.

A. Fast twitch
B. Ectomorph
C. European
D. Mesomorph

32. There are three different fiber types, all present in each muscle. They are the:

A. Pennate, Bi-Pennate and Fusiform.
B. Fast, long and short
C. Endomorph, Ectomorph and Mesomorph
D. None of the above

33. Lifting heavier weight between 1-12 repetitions maximum, results in larger gains and is attributed to fast twitch muscle fibers.

TRUE
FALSE

34. All three muscle fiber types automatically change from one to another depending on the actual routine.

TRUE
FALSE

35. ______________ training is still the best known exercise method for burning calories and losing fat.
A. High volume
B. Low volume
C. Isometric

D. Aquatic

36. Overall, high intensity, low volume exercise is paramount to gaining muscle mass.

TRUE

FALSE

37. ______________ literally means that blood has pumped into the muscles that have been training.

A. Ripped

B. Adrenaline

C. The Pump

D. Tear

38. In a common weight loss situation, it is important for your client to be aware that calories are NOT burning off in the hour following their session.

TRUE

FALSE

39. Saturated and trans fats are known as the:

A. Bad fats

B. Good fats

C. Carb adductors

D. None of the above

40. LDL or "bad" cholesterol builds up inside arteries and can lead to heart disease and stroke.

TRUE

FALSE

41. ____________ are both organic and can be ingested. They are vital to life preservation and can be found in most foods. They support various bodily functions, including all systems.

A. Water

B. Antioxidants

C. Legumes

D. Vitamins and minerals

42. Potassium is the third most abundant mineral in the body and is considered an electrolyte.

TRUE

FALSE

43. A diet pill can only replace will power in the gym during illness, sickness or whenever a person is unable to exercise.

TRUE

FALSE

44. This helps prevent leg, back and knee injuries and is useful for beginners, senior citizens and women who are pregnant:

A. Low impact aerobics
B. High step aerobics
C. High impact aerobics
D. Low volume aerobics

45. If the lower back looks too arched or concaved, the muscles of the lower back are doing too much work. In contrast, if their lower back is convex or at least flattened, you may notice bent knees.

TRUE

FALSE

46. High volume training is:

A. High intensity
B. Low intensity
C. Best for muscle hypertrophy
D. All of the above

47. A set is the number of times your client will lift and lower weight in the course of one exercise.

TRUE

FALSE

48. If your clients are interested in losing weight or toning, they should use heavy weight and perform at least 12-25 reps per set.

TRUE

FALSE

49. Chest exercises include:

A. Dumbbell flyes

B. Hammer curls

C. Squats

D. One arm dumbbell row

50. Bent Knee Raises primarily train the thighs.

TRUE

FALSE

51. The average percentage of body fat for men is 8-12% and 12-16% for women.

TRUE

FALSE

52. Aerobic literally means _______ and includes any type of exercise, usually performed at lower to moderate intensity levels.

A. High volume

B. No oxygen

C. Fitness

D. With oxygen

53. The physical and/or psychological capacity to bear hardship or stress is called:

A. Endurance

B. Focus

C. micronutrient

D. None of the above

54. Fast twitch muscles are best trained using _______ weight.

A. Heavier

B. No

C. Lighter weight

D. Isokinetic

55. Proper head posture will result from practicing keeping the head held:

A. Eyes towards floor

B. Straight up

C. Side to side

D. In hand

56. It is not necessary to enroll in an aerobics class in conjunction with studying this manual.

TRUE

FALSE

57. During ball crunches, make sure your clients lock their hands behind their neck for support.

TRUE

FALSE

58. If someone becomes fatigued or dizzy, have them:

A. Walk around in the room in a circle

B. Front kick

C. Stop

D. Speak up

59. Make sure you <u>never</u> use your client's wrist to check pulse count.

TRUE

FALSE

60. With any punch, power emanates from using the hips and pivoting feet.

TRUE

FALSE

61. All diet and exercise programs start within each individual, not from external sources.

TRUE

FALSE

62. When playing music during peak training, the tempo should be somewhere between __________ BPM.

A. 80-100

B. 150-185

C. 100-150

D. Over 327

63. At first, each client should have no more than 5 aerobics classes per week.

TRUE

FALSE

64. Running, martial arts, kickboxing aerobics, step aerobics, advanced Pilates, power walking, swimming, bicycling, and aerobic dancing, are all considered forms of aerobic exercise.

TRUE
FALSE

65. When focusing on Obliques, have clients perform a crunch, only this time turning their elbows up and over towards the opposite side.

TRUE
FALSE

66. Step Aerobics utilizes stepping up and down from a raised surface (stairs, stepper, Bosu).

TRUE
FALSE

67. Oxygen helps to burn fat and glucose in order to produce:

A. Adenosine
B. Triphosphate
C. Both A&B

D. None of the above

68. Have your clients wear:

A. Sneakers
B. Light weight clothing
C. Jewelry
D. A&B only

69. During the cool down phase, your clients can march in place and then have them follow you around in a circle while jogging.

TRUE
FALSE

70. ______________ is the capability of withstanding stress without injury; adapting to physical or mental modification.

A. Patience
B. Bravery
C. Exercise
D. Flexibility

71. Cardiovascular is physical performance involving the heart and blood vessels, causing a temporary increase in heart rate.

TRUE

FALSE

72. _______________ acts as the brain's file cabinet.

A. Unconscious mind

B. Femur

C. Synapse

D. None of the above

73. Aerobic exercise primarily incorporates:

A. Heavy weights

B. Added dietary protein

C. Lifting a TV set

D. None of the above

74. Cutting out carbs is the safest way to lose weight.

TRUE

FALSE

75. I'm ready to help make a difference in people's lives.

TRUE

FALSE

ESSAY SECTION

A young couple comes to you for training. "Jimmy" is a 25 year old man looking to lose 15 lbs and tone up. "Cassie" wants to gain 10 lb of muscle mass. Detail your plan for each person, totaling 250 words *collectively*. If you use a quote, make sure to site each one (directly next to). Plagiarizing will result in automatic failure. Both grammar and word count are mandatory.

FINAL EXAM FOR

Sports Nutrition Consultant Certification Course

This test contains multiple choice and true/false questions (50 total points) as well as an essay (50 total points). Make sure you have studied the book thoroughly before taking this exam. Simply skimming the text for answers will only hinder your confidence as a consultant and may present dangers to your client.

FULL NAME:
MAILING ADDRESS:
PHONE NUMBER:
EMAIL ADDRESS:

(Choose the Most Appropriate Answer)

1. Amino Acids are the:

A. Essential fatty acids

B. Digestive enzymes

C. Building blocks of protein

D. None Of The Above

2. When setting up a legal business structure, you will need:

A. Corporate press pass

B. $30,000 in capital

C. A tax identification number

D. Someone to co-sign a lease

3. The nutrients that together provide the majority of metabolic energy to an organism are called:

A. Micronutrients

B. Macronutrients

C. Vitamins

D. Glycemic Index

4. _________ provides the suggested amounts to consume daily.

A. RDA

B. FDA

C. DBA

D. None of the above

5. There is no better method than consuming low levels of saturated fats and cholesterol than the:

A. Allergy diet

B. Fasting diet

C. Low carb diet

D. Low fat diet

6. Tyrosine can be manufactured in the body, therefore it is a:

A. Essential amino acid

B. Non-essential amino acid

C. DFA

D. Both A & C

7. Vitamin E:

A. Self-absorbs

B. Taken in large amounts

C. Neutralizes free radicals

D. Found in California

8. Carbohydrates are made up of compounds
containing_________
and the types include_________

A. Carbon/sugars

B. Hydrogen/water

C. Starches/air

D. None of the above

9. To add muscle mass, clients should consume more:

A. Fat

B. Beer

C. Protein

D. Vitamins

10. A strong marketing plan should include:

A. Webdesign
B. Business cards
C. Ads in papers
D. All of the above.

11. The Glycemic Index is the measure of how the food your client eats affects their blood sugar levels.

TRUE
FALSE

12. Vegetarians tend to lack the B complex vitamins which can only be found in animal foods.

TRUE
FALSE

13. Amino Acids are the basic building blocks of proteins.

TRUE
FALSE

14. Protein contains 9 calories per gram and has the most calories of all macronutrients.

TRUE

FALSE

15. When consuming meat and poultry, always buy fresh and cook it thoroughly. Frying, stir frying and microwaving are the best methods of cooking.

TRUE

FALSE

16. Nutrition is the process of nourishing or being nourished by which an organism assimilates food and uses it for growth, health and maintenance.

TRUE

FALSE

17. Iron helps the blood and muscles deliver oxygen to every body cell, and it removes carbon dioxide from them.

TRUE

FALSE

18 In the Cyclical Diet, where vitamin C is increased along with the bioflavinoid quercetin, on the first day, the person is expected to fast and each following day, certain foods are

added back into the diet.

TRUE

FALSE

19. Average body fat for women should be between 8-12 %.
TRUE
FALSE

20. The most important attribute a sports nutritionist can have, is the ability to observe.

TRUE

FALSE

21. "Saxon" is a 26 year old male who is desperately trying to add 20 lbs of muscle mass. He exercises correctly, but his body still does change. Which of the following would *best* suit his needs?

A. Eating more food
B. Increasing the amount of protein
C. Adding Creatine to his regimen
D. None of the above

22. The most common scenario you will encounter is a

person trying to lose weight and tone up. "Balthazar" is a healthy 55 year old woman who is ready to give up dieting after years of trying different methods. Which of the following would *not* be appropriate for her needs?

A. Cutting out all carbs
B. Cutting down on calories
C. Baking foods instead of frying
D. Exercise

23. ______________ is the process of nourishing or being nourished by which an organism assimilates food and uses it for growth, health and maintenance.

A. Exfoliation
B. Low fat diet
C. Nutrition
D. All of the above

24. Macronutrients include alcohol and organic acids.

TRUE
FALSE

25. ______________ comes from the Greek Protas meaning "of primary importance."

A. Protein

B. Energy

C. Biotin

D. Health

26. Disaccharides are comprised of:

A. Fats

B. Sucrose

C. Fatty Acids

D. None of the above

27. Unsaturated fats are considered the "good fats."

TRUE

FALSE

28. The average 2 liter bottle of soda contains 200 calories per serving.

TRUE

FALSE

29. Calories are considered macronutrients.

TRUE

FALSE

30. ___________ are considered Micronutrients because, in comparison with Macronutrients, they are needed by the body in smaller amounts.

A. Fats

B. Tomatoes

C. Grains

D. Vitamins

31. ___________ are vital to life preservation and can be found in most foods. They support various bodily functions, including all systems.

A. Vitamins

B. Minerals

C. Starches

D. A&B only

32. Vitamin D's main function is helping Calcium and Phosphorous absorption.

TRUE

FALSE

33. Chrysanthemum Parthenium is also known as:

A. Niacin

B. Carrot

C. Feverfew

D. Sugar Absorption

34. People taking blood thinning medicines, such as aspirin should limit their intake of ______________.

A. Vitamin K

B. Carbohydrates

C. Vitamin B6

D. All of the above

35. This water-soluble vitamin and is one of 8 members of the B Complex Family and assists in the prevention of neural tube defects in fetuses.

A. Niacin

B. Biotin

C. Folic Acid

D. Citrus

36. ______________ are considered a miracle for the human body. They can help prevent heart disease, lower bad cholesterol levels and control blood pressure.

A. Fish Oils

B. Antidepressants

C. One a day vitamins

D. Flax seeds

37. Iron helps the blood and muscles deliver oxygen to every body cell, and it replaces carbon dioxide with white blood cells.

TRUE

FALSE

38. Zinc is a component of over 200 enzymes, most of which are involved in protein and DNA synthesis.

TRUE

FALSE

39. _____________ is used as a dietary supplement for better water-solubility to proteins in neutral solution. It is also considered essential to the diet of children for optimum rates of growth.

A. Glucose

B. Arginine

C. Amino Fuel

D. Turkey

40. If your client is concerned about adding water weight, let them know it's not from ____________.

A. Cola

B. Lemonade

C. Water

D. Grape juice

41. <u>Miso</u>, <u>Navy beans</u>, <u>Pinto beans</u>, <u>Soybeans</u>, <u>Tempeh</u>, and <u>Tofu</u> all fall into the ________________ category.

A. Vegetables

B. Seeds

C. B Complex Vitamins

D. Legumes

42. Fish, such as salmon, has less saturated fat, cholesterol and essential fatty acids the body uses to function properly.

TRUE

FALSE

43. People who suffer from food allergies should consult a psychologist to rule out psychosomatic origins before attributing their allergies to digestive malfunction.

TRUE

FALSE

44. Complex carbohydrates that break down slowly have a higher glycemic index.

TRUE
FALSE

45. BPM is short for:

A. Breaks Per Myositus
B. Balanced Protein Absorption
C. Body to Fat Percentage
D. Beats Per Minute

46. Standard target heart rate during exercise:

A. Age 18-30, 120-146 BPM
B. Age 31-40, 93-138 BPM
C. Age 41-50, 88-131 RDA
D. None of the above

47. For people worried about pesticides, ______________ are all natural.

A. Organic foods
B. Frozen foods

C. Canned fruits

D. Wrapped candy bars

48. The average percentage of body fat for men is 8-12% and 12-16% for women.

TRUE

FALSE

49. When the body is lacking in proper nutrients (i.e. carbohydrates), it will need to tap into muscles as an energy source.

TRUE

FALSE

50. I am ready to assist people who are serious about taking better care of themselves.

TRUE

FALSE

ESSAY SECTION

A father and daughter come to you for advice. "Ernie" is a 50 year old man looking to lose

15 lbs and has trouble laying off of fast food. "Nina" wants to gain 10 lb of muscle mass for an upcoming movie role. Detail your plan for each person, totaling 500 words *collectively*. If you use a quote, make sure to site each one (directly next to). Plagiarizing will result in automatic failure. Both grammar and word count are mandatory. Good luck!

FINAL EXAM FOR

Advanced Personal Trainer Certification Course

This test contains multiple choice and true/false questions (50 total points) as well as an essay (50 total points). Make sure you have studied the entire book thoroughly before taking this exam (this is an accumulative exam based on *both* levels of personal trainer certification- advanced candidates should be proficient in our level one material). Simply skimming the text for answers will only hinder your confidence as a trainer and may present dangers to your client. A grade of 85%

is required for passing. Work hard and **GOOD LUCK!**

FULL NAME:
MAILING ADDRESS:
PHONE NUMBER:
EMAIL ADDRESS:
(Choose the Most Appropriate Answer)

1. When training your abdominal muscles, it is important to isolate the different sections (i.e. upper and lower abs) by using different exercises.

TRUE
FALSE

2. Lifting heavier weight between 12-25 repetitions results in larger gains and is the most beneficial formula for building muscle mass.

TRUE
FALSE

3. A good motto for an advanced personal trainer to endorse is:

A. Train, don't strain
B. Weights get dates
C. No pain, no gain
D. None of the above

4. In Yoga, _______________ are comprised of several combinations of stretching and breathing.

A. Sets
B. Asanas
C. Positions
D. Parvatasan

5. Anaerobic movement requires oxygen, which occurs during high volume, high intensity exercise.

TRUE
FALSE

6. Boddhidharma is noted for:

A. Kung Fu
B. Bringing Yoga to Japan
C. Pilates Mountain Pose

D. None of the above

7. The most common scenario you will encounter is a person trying to lose weight and tone up. Let's assume "Margarita" is a healthy 38 year old woman. Which of the following can she use to attain her goals?

A. Step aerobics
B. Weight training
C. Low fat diet
D. All of the above

8. A person with shorter tendons and longer biceps will acheive better results compared to someone with longer tendons and shorter biceps:

TRUE
FALSE

9. Which of the following *isn't* a Pilates Technique:

A. The Americana
B. The Roll Up
C. Bridge
D. Ballerina Arms

10. Aerobic literally means _________ and includes any type of exercise, usually performed at lower to moderate intensity levels.

A. High volume

B. No oxygen

C. Fitness

D. With oxygen

11. There are various forms of yoga, but four of the most popular types are: Hatha Yoga, Strength Yoga, Iyengar and Bikram Yoga.

TRUE

FALSE

12. Fast twitch muscles are best trained using _________ weight.

A. Heavier

B. No

C. Lighter

D. Isokinetic

13. Proper head posture will result from practicing keeping the head held:

A. Eyes towards floor

B. Straight up

C. Side to side

D. In hand

14. It is not necessary to enroll in an aerobics class in conjunction with studying this manual.

TRUE

FALSE

15. During ball crunches, make sure your clients lock their hands behind their neck for support.

TRUE

FALSE

16. If someone becomes fatigued or dizzy, have them:

A. Walk around in the room in a circle

B. Front kick

C. Stop

D. Speak up

17. Make sure you <u>never</u> use your client's wrist to check pulse count.

TRUE

FALSE

18. With any punch, power emanates from using the hips and pivoting feet.

TRUE
FALSE

19. <u>Synarthrosis</u> permits flexibility, such as in the elbows.

TRUE
FALSE

20. When playing music during peak training, the tempo should be somewhere between __________ BPM.

A. 80-100
B. 150-185
C. 100-150
D. Over 327

21. At first, each client should have no more than 5 aerobics classes per week.

TRUE
FALSE

22. Running, martial arts, kickboxing aerobics, step aerobics, advanced Pilates, power walking, swimming, bicycling, and aerobic dancing, are all considered forms of aerobic exercise.

TRUE
FALSE

23. When focusing on Obliques, have clients perform a crunch, only this time turning their elbows up and over towards the opposite side.

TRUE
FALSE

24. Step Aerobics utilizes stepping up and down from a raised surface (stairs, stepper, Bosu).

TRUE
FALSE

25. Oxygen helps to burn fat and glucose in order to produce:

A. Adenosine
B. Triphosphate
C. Both A&B
D. None of the above

26. Unlike free weights, where gravity is used as the antagonist, _____________________ use consistent tension that makes movement feel awkward initially.

A. Isokinetic machines

B. Dumbells

C. Resistance bands

D. All of the above

27. During the cool down phase, your clients can march in place and then have them follow you around in a circle while jogging.

TRUE

FALSE

28. _____________ is the capability of withstanding stress without injury; adapting to physical or mental modification.

A. Patience

B. Bravery

C. Exercise

D. Flexibility

29. Cardiovascular is physical performance involving the heart and blood vessels, causing a temporary increase in heart rate.

TRUE

FALSE

30. Weight loss = high volume, low intensity exercise. Muscle building = high intensity, low volume exercise.

TRUE

FALSE

31. When setting up a legal business structure, you will need:

A. Corporate press pass
B. $30,000 in capital
C. A tax identification number
D. Someone to co-sign a lease

32. The muscles of the neck are called the:

A. Neck flexors
B. Sterno Mastoids
C. Gastrocnemous
D. Quadriceps

33. Charles Atlas favored this form of training and developed a group of exercises including these techniques.

A. Isometrics

B. Pilates

C. Static

D. Isontonic

34. Protein contains 9 calories per gram and has the most calories of all macronutrients.

TRUE

FALSE

35. High volume training is:

A. High intensity

B. Low intensity

C. Performed with loud music

D. Requires "train to failure" approach

36. The Ectomorph body type is:

A. Naturally muscular

B. Usually thin

C. Obese in certain areas

D. Both A & C

37. ___________________ begin at the pelvic bone and join at intervals along the extent of the femur.

A. Thigh bones

B. Adductor muscles

C. Brachii

D. None of the above

38. This muscle of the abdomen lies underneath all the other abdominal muscles and wraps sideways around the entire abdominal area.

A. Transverse Abdominus

B. Hip flexions

C. Humerus

D. Tibia

39. Joints allow movement and provide structural support to bones, tendons, muscles, and ligaments.

TRUE

FALSE

40. Ligaments are comprised of strands of <u>collagen</u> fibers.

TRUE

FALSE

41. The Cranium is also known as the:

A. Collarbone

B. Chest plate

C. Clavicle

D. Skull

42. The Ischis is the technical term for the spinal column.

TRUE

FALSE

43. ___________________ exercises are performed similar to regular methods, only they're positioned differently.

A. Isokinetic

B. Static

C. Resistance bands

D. All of the above

44. The Fibula is a large, triangular <u>bone</u> which works in conjunction with the *Femur* and protects the knee joint.

TRUE

FALSE

45. The three structural classifications of joints are the Fibrous Joint, Cartilaginous Joint and Synovial Joint.

TRUE

FALSE

46. With clients on their hands and knees, ask them to wrap a band around their right foot. Holding the handles (with hands facing floor), have them extend their right leg straight back, squeezing the glutes in a even motion. Have them hold for a second, return slowly and repeat with their left leg. This exercise is called a:

A. Kick back
B. Isotonic heel flex
C. Cat stretch
D. Glute Kick

47. Isometric training is an effective system of <u>exercise</u> where the practitioner contracts his/her muscle without any movement in the joint.

TRUE

FALSE

48. Isokinetics is an exercise performed with a particular machine so that depending on how much force is exerted, the movement takes place at varied speeds.

TRUE

FALSE

49. Joints are anotomically located in these groups:

A. Cranium
B. Knees
C. Sinus Cavity
D. Collar bone

50. I will use the advanced personal training information I've learned to show off my expertise over my clients.

TRUE
FALSE

ESSAY SECTION

A father and daughter come to you for training. "Adam" is a 50 year old man looking to lose 15 lbs and tone up. "Emily" has entered a bodybuilding contest and wants to gain 10 lb of muscle mass. Detail your plan for each person, totaling 500 words *collectively*. If you use a quote, make sure to site each one (directly next to).

Plagiarizing will result in automatic failure. Both grammar and word count are mandatory. Good luck!

TOP TIER EXAM ANSWER KEY

Personal Trainer Certification

1. T
2. C
3. B
4. A
5. F
6. B
7. B
8. C
9. C
10. D
11. F
12. F
13. A
14. T
15. F
16. F
17. D
18. D
19. F
20. C
21. T
22. F
23. B
24. T
25. F
26. A

27. T
28. D
29. A
30. A
31. D
32. A
33. T
34. T
35. A
36. T
37. C
38. F
39. A
40. T
41. D
42. T
43. F
44. A
45. T
46. B
47. F
48. F
49. A
50. F
51. T
52. D
53. A
54. A
55. B
56. F
57. F
58. C
59. F
60. T
61. T
62. C

63. F
64. T
65. T
66. T
67. C
68. D
69. T
70. D
71. T
72. A
73. D
74. F
75. T

TOP TIER EXAM ANSWER KEY
Sports Nutrition Certification

1. C
2. C
3. B
4. A
5. D
6. B
7. C
8. A
9. C
10. D
11. T
12. T
13. T
14. F
15. F
16. T
17. T
18. F

19. F
20. T
21. B
22. A
23. C
24. T
25. T
26. B
27. T
28. T
29. F
30. D
31. D
32. T
33. C
34. A
35. C
36. A
37. F
38. T
39. B
40. C
41. D
42. F
43. F
44. F
45. D
46. B
47. A
48. T
49. T
50. T

TOP TIER EXAM ANSWER KEY
Advanced Personal Trainer Certification

1. F
2. F
3. A
4. B
5. F
6. A
7. D
8. T
9. A
10. D
11. F
12. A
13. B
14. F
15. F
16. C
17. F
18. T
19. F
20. C
21. F
22. T
23. T
24. T
25. C
26. C
27. T
28. D
29. T
30. T
31. C
32. B
33. A
34. F
35. B

36. B
37. B
38. A
39. T
40. T
41. D
42. T
43. C
44. F
45. T
46. D
47. T
48. F
49. F
50. F

Michael Jonathan Rocco, PhD is a husband, author, producer, musician, 3rd Dan Black Belt Martial Artist, Certified Personal Trainer (CPT), podcaster, and cat lover. He lives on Long Island, New York with his wife Kristina and 8 cats.

Baechle, Thomas R, and National Strength & Conditioning Association (U.S. *Essentials of Strength Training and Conditioning*. Champaign, Il, Human Kinetics, 1994.

Bean, Anita, and James Cracknell. *Sports Nutrition*. Londres, A & C Black, Cop, 2009.

Carnegie, Dale, and Dorothy Carnegie. *How to Stop Worrying and Start Living*. New York, Simon And Schuster, 1984.

Connors, Ed, and Gold's Gym. *The Gold's Gym Encyclopedia of Bodybuilding*. Lincolnwood, Ill., Contemporary Books, 1998.

Frédéric Delavier. *Strength Training Anatomy*. Champaign (Il), Human Kinetics, 2010.

English Sports Council. *Sports Nutrition*. London, Sports Council, 1996.

Goodman, Jonathan. *Ignite the Fire : The Secrets to Building a Successful Personal Training Career*. North Charleston, S.C., Createspace, 2014.

Hoffer, Abram, and Andrew W Saul. *Orthomolecular Medicine for Everyone : Megavitamin Therapeutics for Families and Physicians.* Laguna Beach, Ca, Basic Health, 2008.

Kotler, Philip, and Gary Armstrong. *Principles of Marketing.* Hoboken, Pearson Higher Education, 2018.

Mackay, Jenny. *Sports Nutrition.* Farmington Hills, Mich., Lucent Books, A Part Of Gale, Cengage Learning, 2015.

Neff, Fred, and James E Reid. *Basic Jujitsu Handbook.* Minneapolis, Lerner, 1976.

Morihei Ueshiba, and John Stevens. *The Art of Peace.* Boulder, Shambhala, 2018.

Wade, Jennifer. *Personal Training : Individual Fitness Programs & Training Plans for Every Body Type.* New York, Sterling Pub. Co, 1998.

8 Principles, *190*
Abdominals, *55, 90*
absorption, *67*
Adductor Muscles, *160*
Advanced Anatomy, *158*
ADVANCED PERSONAL TRAINER CERTIFICATION, *157*
Aerobic, *51, 96*
Aerobic Kickboxing, *178*
aerobics, *186*
Aerobics, *96, 98*
aerobics class, *103*
AIDS, *117*
Alanine, *125*
Albert Einstein, *142*
Alcohol, *68*
Alignment, *190*
Allergy Diet, *144*
Amino Acids, *124*
Amphiarthrosis, *162*
Anaerobic, *51*
anatomy, *159*
Anatomy, *158*
Angled Calf Raise, *89*
Antioxidants, *118*

Arginine, *125*
arm scissors, *101*
Arms, *74*
as *cardio kickboxing*, *178*
Asanas, *201*
ascorbic acid, *117*
Assessment Tests, *72*
AUC, *145*
autoimmune diseases, *121*
B complex Vitamins, *66, 117*
B Complex Vitamins, *66, 117*
<u>**Back**</u>, *87*
balance, *76*
Balance, *51, 202*
Ball Crunches, *90*
Ballerina Arms, *194*
Barbell Bench press, *82*
Barbell Bench Press, *82*
Basic Fighting Stance, *180*
Basic Nutrition, *63*
Beans & Legumes, *134*
Believe, *28*
Bench Dips, *86*
Bench Press, *82*
Bends, *202*
Bent Knee Raises, *91*
Bernh, *119*

Bicep Curl, *171*
Biceps, *54, 85*
Biceps Femorus, *56*
Bikram Yoga, *200*
bioflavinoid quercetin, *144*
Biotin, *119*
bi-pennate, 58
BJJ, *210*
blood glucose levels, *145*
blood pressure, *121*
Boddhidharma, *205*
body, *76*
body fat, *92*
Body Types, *56*
bodybuilders, *173*
Bone Anatomy, 165
Bosu, *99, 169*
boxing, *185*
BPM, *79, 98, 147, 184*
Brachialis, 55
brain, *121*
Break Falls, *220*
Breastbone, 166
***Breathing**, 91, 190*
Brevis, *160*
Bridge, *195*
Bridge on Exercise Ball, *195*
Bruce Lee, *207*

Buddhism, *198*
Business Cards, *9*
Buttocks, 76
calcium, *122*
calf, *168*
Calfbone, 168
Calories, *64, 116*
Calves, 77
cancer, *117*
Canned foods, *148*
carbohydrates, *145*
Carbohydrates, *65, 115*
carbon dioxide, *68*
carbs, *65, 140*
cardio kickboxing, 178
Cardiovascular, *52*
Carpals, 167
Cartilaginous Joint, *162*
Case Studies, *151*
CASE STUDIES, *104*
Cat Stretch, *75, 197*
C-Curve, *196*
Centering, *191*
cereal, *120*
Charles Atlas, *173*
<u>**Chest**</u>, *82*
Chest Press, *170*
Chin Gempin, *208*
cholesterol, *119, 143*

Cholesterol, *64*
Chrysanthemum
    parthenium, *119*
Circuit Training, *179*
Class Designs, *183*
Clavicle, *166*
Coccyx, *167*
Coenzyme Q10, *120*
Collarbone, *166*
Concentration, *190*
Conclusion, *112*
Contents, *4*
cool down phase, *102*
Coordination, *51*
Co-ordination, *191*
Cranium, *166*
Creatine, *70, 127*
Cross punch, *182*
Crunches, *90*
D.B.A., *7*
D.B.A. or *Doing Business
    As*, *7*
dairy, *120*
Deltoids, *54*
depression, *121*
Determination, *53*
Diarthrosis, *162*
Diet Theories, *140*
dizzy, *103*
DNA synthesis, *124*

Dumbbell Bench Press,
    82
Dumbbell Flyes, *83*
Dumbbell Lunges, *89*
Dumbbell Squats, *88*
Ectomorphs, *57*
eggs, *124*
Elastic Band Press, *83*
Elbow Strikes, *183*
electrolyte, *123*
Endomorphs, *57*
Endurance, *52*
energy, *122*
epididymis, *38*
essential amino acid,
    126
Etiquette, *215*
exam, *226*
Exercise, *48*
Exercise Routine, *80*
exercises, *168*
Explosiveness, *51*
Extension, *183*
Extensor Carpi, *55*
fast twitch fiber, *59*
Fat, *64*
Fats, *116*
fat-soluble, *118*
FDA, *144*
Femur, *167*
Feverfew, *118*

Fibrous Joint, *162*
Fibula, *168*
fish, *123*
Fish Oil, *121*
fitness trainer, *13*
flexibility, *72*
Flexibility, *51*
Flowing Movements, *191*
Flyers, *9*
Focus, *52*
Folic Acid, *120*
Food Pyramid, *144*
forced rep, *62*
Forearm Muscles, *55*
Front Dumbbell Raise, *84*
Front Kick, *181*
frozen foods, *148*
Fruits, *132*
fusiform, *58*
Gastrocnemeus, *56*
Gichin Funakoshi, *212*
glucose, *123*
Glutamine, *126*
Glute Kick, *172*
Glutes, *56*
Gluteus Maximus, *56*
Glycemic Index, *145*
Gracie Jiu-Jitsu, *209*
Gracilis, *160*

grains, *120*
Grains, *136*
Hammer Curls, *86*
Hamstrings, *56, 76*
Hand, *167*
Hatha Yoga, *200*
headaches, *119*
health, *124*
health questionnaire, *6*
Health Questionnaire, *104, 222*
Healthy Foods, *71, 128*
Heart Rate, *78, 146*
heartbeat, *123*
Helpful Tips, *92*
Herbs & Spices, *137*
High intensity exercises, *61*
High volume exercises, *60*
<u>**High-Impact Aerobics**</u>, *99*
hip flexion, *160*
hip flexor, *74*
Hook Punch, *182*
Humerus, *160, 166*
hypertrophy, *62*
hypotrophy, *121*
IBS, *39*
Iliacus, *159*

Iliopsoas, *160*
Iliopsoas Muscle, *159*
immune system, *122*
Incline Dumbbell Press, *83*
Infra-Spranatis, *55*
Inner Thigh Stretch, *197*
insurance, *8*
Inversion, *203*
Iron, *68*, *122*
Ischis, *166*
Isokinetic training, *176*
Isokinetics, *175*
Isometric Calf Raise, *175*
Isometric Push Ups, *174*
Isometric Rows, *174*
Isometric Shoulder Raise, *174*
Isometric Squats, *174*
Isometric Training, *172*
Isometrics, *173*
Isotonic, *80*
Isotonic Training, *80*
Jab Punch, *182*
Jeet Kune Do, *207*
Jigoro Kano, *210*
joints, *161*

Joints, *161*
Joseph H. Pilates, *188*
Judo, *210*, *211*
juices, *123*
Jujitsu, *207*
Karate, *211*, *212*
kickboxing, *215*
Kickboxing Aerobics, *178*
Kickboxing Pointers, *185*
Kickboxing Techniques, *179*
knee, *101*
knee raises, *161*
Knee Variations, *183*
Kneecap, *168*
krisitna rocco, *2*
Kristina Rocco, 2
Kung Fu, *206*
Latissimus Dorsi, *54*
Lats, *54*
Legs, *88*
legumes, *121*
Ligaments, *163*
Local Papers, *11*
Longus, *160*
Lotus Pose, *201*
Low Carbohydrate Diet, *140*
Low Fat Dairy, *134*

Low Fat Diet, *143*
Lower Back, 75
Low-Impact Aerobics, 98
Lumbars, *55*
Lying Dumbbell
   Extensions, *87*
Macronutrients, *114,
   120*
Magnesium, *67, 122*
Magnus, *160*
Marketing, *7, 9*
Martial Arts, *173, 204*
***Martial Arts
   Techniques, 219***
meat, *120*
Meat, *138*
medium twitch fibers,
   59
menadione, *119*
menaquinone, *119*
Mesomorphs, *57*
Metabolism, *52*
Metacarpals, 167
Michael J. Rocco, *282*
Micronutrients, *116*
migraine, *119*
milk, *127*
***Mind Over
   Everything, 12***
Minerals, *65, 117*
mixed martial arts, *204*

MMA, *185, 204*
mobility, *162*
***Motivation**, 12*
Mountain pose, 201
Movie Theaters, *11*
Muay Thai, *214*
Muscle building, *60*
Muscle Fiber, *58*
muscle fiber types, *59*
Muscle Groups, *53*
muscle mass, *61*
music, *100*
Neck, 74
Neutral Spine, *194*
Niacin, *120*
non-essential amino
   acid, *126*
Nutrition, *52, 63, 113*
Nuts & Seeds, *135*
O.P.A.L., *7*
Obliques, *103*
Obloquies, *55*
Omega-3, *121*
One Arm Dumbbell
   Row, *88*
organic, *117*
Organic foods, *148*
Overhead Press, *171*
pancreas, *123*
Pantothenic acid, *119*
Pantothenic Acid, *121*

Patanjali, *198*
Patella, *168*
peanuts, *122*
Pecs, *54*
Pectineus, *160*
Pectoralis, *54*
Pelvis, *167*
pennate, *58*
Performance Supplements, *70, 127*
personal trainer, *53*
PERSONAL TRAINER CERTIFICATION, *12*
Personal training, *63*
Personal Training, *63*
Phalanges, *167*
Phenylalanine, *126*
phosphorus, *122*
phylloquinone, *119*
phytochemicals, *116*
Pilates, *187, 193, 198*
Pilates Techniques, *193*
Placemat Advertising, *11*
Positions, *201*
Postcards, *9*
Potassium, *68, 123*

poultry, *120*
Poultry, *138*
Poultry & Meat, *138*
Power Yoga, *200*
Protein, *69, 114*
Protein Shake, *71, 127*
Psoas, *159*
pulldowns, *169*
Punch, *182*
Pyrethrum parthenium, *119*
Quadriceps, *56*
radial artery, *79*
Radio, *11*
Radius, *167*
RDA, *150*
Rear Delt Row, *170*
Recommended Dietary Allowance, *150*
Rectus Abdominus, *161*
Relaxation, *190, 204*
release form, *6*
Release Form, *224*
repetition, *179*
reps, *100*
Resistance bands, *168*
Resistance Bands, *168*
Rhomboids, *55*

Riboflavin, *121*
Rotational Diet, *144*
Rotator Cuff, *55*
Roundhouse Kick, *181*
Sacrum, *167*
Samadhi, *198*
SAMPLE FORMS, *222*
saturated, *116*
Scapula, *166*
seafood, *124*
Seafood, *132*
Seated Dumbbell Curls, *85*
Seated Dumbbell Press, *84*
Selenium, *69*, *123*
serotonin, *120*
set, *179*
Set Up, *7*
Sheershasana, *204*
Shoulder Shrugs, *85*
Shoulders, *75*, *84*
Side Bridge, *175*
Side Dumbbell Raise, *85*
Side Kick, *181*
side steps, *100*
Side Steps, *172*
Six Pack, *55*
six-pack, *161*

Skull, *165*
slow twitch fibers, *58*
Sodium, *70*, *124*
soybeans, *120*
Speed, *52*
spina bifida, *120*
spinal column, *166*
Spinal Erectors, *55*
SPORTS NUTRITION CONSULTANT CERTIFICATION, *113*
Squat, *180*
Squats, *171*
Stamina, *191*
Standing Barbell Curls, *86*
Static, *172*
<u>**Step Aerobics**</u>, *99*
stepper, *101*
Sterno Mastoids, *53*
Sternum, *166*
stomach, *55*
Stomach crunches, *160*
Strength, *51*
Stretch, *197*
stretching, *74*
Sub-Scapularis, *55*
Super-Spranatis, *55*
Supine, *203*

Supplements, *143*

Sweeteners, *139*

Synarthrosis, *162, 267*

Synovial Joint, *162*

Tae Kwon Do, *213*

Tailbone, 167

Tarsus, *168*

Tendon, *164*

***Tendons**, 163*

Teres Major and Minor, 55

The Hundred, *195*

***The Powerhouse**, 189*

The Roll Up, *194*

The Saw, *195*

The Spine, *192*

The Swan, *196*

The Torso, *192*

Thiamine, *121*

Thighbone, 167

Thighs, 76

Tibia, *168*

***To Believe Is To See, 28*

Toe Raises, *180*

torso, *192*

Torso Twist, *183*

Train, don't strain, 94

trainer, *80*

trans fats, *116*

Transverse Abdominus, *161*

Trapezius, *53*

Treadmill, *91*

Triceps, *54, 86*

Triceps Brachii, *160*

Tryptophan, *126*

TV, *11*

Twist Crunches, *90*

Twists, *203*

Tyrosine, *126*

unconscious mind, *15*

upper back, *73*

Vegan, *142*

Vegetables, *129*

Vegetarian, *142*

vegetarians, *143*

Vertebra, *166*

Vitamin A, *66, 117*

Vitamin C, *66, 117*

Vitamin D, *66, 118*

Vitamin E, *67, 118*

Vitamin K, *119*

Vitamins, *65, 117*

Volume vs. Intensity Training, *60*

water, *128*

water-soluble, *121*

Website, *10*

Weight, *80*

Weight loss, *60, 193*

Weight Loss, *127*
Weight Loss Supplements, *71*
Welcome, *5*
whey, *127*
Wide Grip Pull-Down, *88*

Wrist Bones, *167*
yeast, *120*
Yoga, *173*, *198*
Yoga Poses, *201*
Zinc, *70*, *124*